VINCENT J. MANDRACCHIA, DPM, MS
CONSULTING EDITOR

CLINICS IN PODIATRIC MEDICINE AND SURGERY

Diabetes Mellitus

GARY PETER JOLLY, DPM, FACFAS
THOMAS ZGONIS, DPM, GUEST EDITORS

VOLUME 20 • NUMBER 4 • OCTOBER 2003

W.B. SAUNDERS COMPANY
A Division of Elsevier Inc.
PHILADELPHIA LONDON TORONTO MONTREAL SYDNEY TOKYO

W.B. SAUNDERS COMPANY
A Division of Elsevier Inc.

The Curtis Center • Independence Square West • Philadelphia, Pennsylvania 19106

http://www.theclinics.com

CLINICS IN PODIATRIC MEDICINE AND SURGERY
October 2003
Editor: Karen Sorensen

Volume 20, Number 4
ISSN 0891-8422

Reprints. For copies of 100 or more of articles in this publication, please contact the Commercial Reprints Department, Elsevier Inc., 360 Park Avenue South, New York, New York 10010-1710 Tel.: (212) 633-3813, Fax: (212) 633-3820, e-mail: reprints@elsevier.com

Clinics in Podiatric Medicine and Surgery (ISSN 0891-8422) is published quarterly by W.B. Saunders Company. Corporate and editorial Offices: The Curtis Center, Independence Square West, Philadelphia, PA 19106–3399. Accounting and circulation offices: 6277 Sea Harbor Drive, Orlando, FL 32887–4800. Periodicals postage paid at Orlando, FL 32862, and additional mailing offices. Subscription prices are $160.00 per year for US individuals, $243.00 per year for US institutions, $80.00 per year for US students and residents, $193.00 per year for Canadian individuals, $294.00 per year for Canadian institutions $215.00 per year for international individuals, $294.00 per year for international institutions and $107.00 per year for Canadian and foreign students/residents. To receive student/resident rate, orders must be accompanied by name of affiliated institution, date of term, and the *signature* of program/residency coordinator on institution letterhead. Orders will be billed at individual rate until proof of status is received. Foreign air speed delivery is included in all *Clinics* subscription prices. All prices are subject to change without notice. POSTMASTER: Send address changes to *Clinics in Podiatric Medicine and Surgery*, W.B. Saunders Company, Periodicals Fulfillment, Orlando, FL 32887-4800. **Customer Service: 1-800-654-2452 (US). From outside of the US, call 1-407-345-1000.**

Clinics in Podiatric Medicine and Surgery is covered in *Index Medicus* and *EMBASE/Excerpta Medica.*

Printed in the United States of America.

CONSULTING EDITOR

VINCENT J. MANDRACCHIA, DPM, MS, Section Chief, Podiatric Surgery, Department of Surgery, Broadlawns Medical Center; and Clinical Professor, Department of Podiatric Medicine and Surgery, College of Podiatric Medicine and Surgery, Des Moines University - Osteopathic Medicine Center, Des Moines, Iowa

GUEST EDITORS

GARY PETER JOLLY, DPM, FACFAS, Clinical Professor of Surgery, Des Moines University, School of Podiatric Medicine and Surgery, Des Moines, Iowa; Director of PGY IV Fellowship in Reconstructive Foot and Ankle Surgery and Chief of Podiatric Surgery, New Britain General Hospital, New Britain, Connecticut; Senior Consultant and Site Director, West Haven VAMC, West Haven, Connecticut

THOMAS ZGONIS, DPM, Postdoctoral Fellow, Department of Orthopedics, Yale School of Medicine, New Haven, Connecticut; Fellow, Reconstructive Foot and Ankle Surgery, and Staff, New Britain General Hospital, New Britain, Connecticut

CONTRIBUTORS

JAMES BERNENE, MD, Chief, Department of Medicine, New Britain General Hospital, New Britain, Connecticut; Professor and Associate Chairman of Medicine, University of Connecticut School of Medicine, Farmington, Connecticut

PETER BLUME, DPM, Assistant Clinical Professor of Orthopedics and Rehabilitation, Yale University School of Medicine; and Director of Limb Salvage, Yale-New Haven Hospital, New Haven, Connecticut

BENJAMIN J. BUREN, DPM, Second Year Podiatric Surgical Resident , West Haven-Yale Podiatric Surgical Residency, West Haven, Connecticut

ROBERT G. FRYKBERG, DPM, MPH, Chief, Podiatry Section, Carl T. Hayden VA Medical Center, Phoenix, Arizona

JOHN M. GIURINI, DPM, Assistant Professor, Department of Surgery, Harvard Medical School; Chief, Division of Podiatry, Beth Israel Deaconess Medical Center, Harvard Medical School, Boston, Massachusetts

DAWN M. GROSSER, MD, Third Year Resident, Department of Orthopaedics and Rehabilitation, Yale University, New Haven, Connecticut

GARY PETER JOLLY, DPM, FACFAS, Clinical Professor of Surgery, Des Moines University, School of Podiatric Medicine and Surgery, Des Moines, Iowa; Director of PGY IV Fellowship in Reconstructive Foot Surgery and Chief of Podiatric Surgery, New Britain General Hospital, New Britain, Connecticut; Senior Consultant and Site Director, West Haven VAMC, West Haven, Connecticut

TAESEUNG LEE, MD, Postdoctoral Fellow in Vascular Surgery, Yale University School of Medicine, New Haven, Connecticut

WILLIAM A. PETIT, Jr, MD, FACP, FACE, Assistant Professor of Clinical Medicine, Yale University School of Medicine, New Haven, Connecticut and University of Connecticut, Farmington, Connecticut; Medical Director, Joslin Diabetes Center Affiliate at New Britain General Hospital, New Britain, Connecticut

VASILIOS POLYZIOS, MD, Chief Orthopaedic Resident, Thriasson General Hospital, Elefsina, Greece

BARRY I. ROSENBLUM, DPM, Assistant Clinical Professor, Department of Surgery, Harvard Medical School; Director, Podiatric Medical Education, Beth Israel Deaconess Medical Center, Boston, Massachusetts

KATHLEEN SATTERFIELD, DPM, Fellow, American College of Foot and Ankle Medicine, Orthopaedics and Medicine, Ellicott City, Maryland; Associate Professor, Department of Orthopaedics, University of Texas Health Science Center at San Antonio, San Antonio, Texas

LEE R. SAYNER, DPM, Resident, Division of Podiatry, Department of Surgery, Beth Israel Deaconess Medical Center; Clinical Fellow in Surgery, Harvard Medical School, Boston, Massachusetts

ENZO J. SELLA, MD, Associate Clinical Professor of Orthopaedic Surgery, Yale University Department of Orthopaedics and Rehabilitation; Co-Director of Foot and Ankle Clinic, Yale New Haven Hospital, New Haven, Connecticut; Connecticut Orthopaedic Specialists, Hamden, Connecticut

BAUER E. SUMPIO, MD, PhD, Professor of Surgery and Radiology, Chief of Vascular Surgery, Yale University School of Medicine, New Haven, Connecticut

RAGHU P. UPENDER, MD, Neurology Consultant, Joslin Diabetes Center Affiliate at New Britain General Hospital, New Britain, Connecticut

THOMAS ZGONIS, DPM, Postdoctoral Fellow, Department of Orthopedics, Yale School of Medicine, New Haven, Connecticut; Fellow, Reconstructive Foot and Ankle Surgery, and Staff, New Britain General Hospital, New Britain, Connecticut

CONTENTS

Foreword xi
Vincent J. Mandracchia

Preface xiii
Gary Peter Jolly and Thomas Zgonis

Diabetes Mellitus and Pharmacological Therapy 635
James Bernene, Thomas Zgonis, and Gary Peter Jolly

Diabetes mellitus can be a devastating lifelong disease if not treated appropriately. The physician and the patient should be aware of both extremes involved with DM: hyperglycemia and hypoglycemia. Enormous advances in the treatment of diabetes have occurred over the past decade and even greater ones can be expected in the future. This article discusses the new drugs, insulin delivery devices, and noninvasive glucose monitoring machines currently available for the treatment of diabetes mellitus.

Diabetic Foot Infections and Antibiotic Therapy 655
Thomas Zgonis, Gary Peter Jolly, Benjamin J. Buren, and Peter Blume

Diabetic foot infections are the most common cause of lower extremity amputations. Diabetic neuropathy, angiopathy, renal disease, and multisystem failure are some of the factors that can lead to a limb or a life-threatening infection and subsequent amputation. Soft tissue or bone infections in diabetics are usually managed surgically, supplemented by antibiotic therapy and vascular reconstruction when appropriate. Aggressive surgical intervention and appropriate antibiotic therapy will reduce the likelihood of major amputations and the duration of hospitalization.

Medical Evaluation and Treatment of Diabetic Peripheral Neuropathy 671
William A. Petit, Jr and Raghu P. Upender

Diabetes mellitus is a major health problem that is expected to become more prevalent over the next few decades. It causes much morbidity and mortality through various macro- and microvascular complications, including diabetic neuropathy. Because treatments options are limited, and frequently unsatisfactory, prevention of diabetic foot complications becomes even more imperative. This article reviews our current understanding of diabetic neuropathy.

Vascular Evaluation and Arterial Reconstruction of the Diabetic Foot 689
Bauer E. Sumpio, Taeseung Lee, and Peter A. Blume

Management of the diabetic foot is often a complex clinical problem. The pathophysiologic mechanisms underlying diabetic foot disease include neuropathy, infection, and ischemia. However, the principles of care are simple, including correction of systemic and local factors. This article discusses clinical evaluation of the diabetic foot and various methods of arterial reconstruction.

Diabetic Foot Ulcerations: Management and Adjunctive Therapy 709
Robert G. Frykberg

Foot ulcerations in individuals who have diabetes mellitus are major risk factors for infection, osteomyelitis, and gangrene. Each of these lesions has consistently been ascertained as a significant risk factor for subsequent lower extremity amputations. A multidisciplinary team approach as been demonstrated as the most successful way to manage and prevent foot lesions in individuals who have diabetes. Such teams provide education, appropriate foot care, and early intervention as key components in their programs, which are focused on amputation prevention. This article reviews the epidemiology, current understanding of the underlying pathophysiology, and treatment rationale for diabetic foot ulcerations. When evidence-based concepts are incorporated into daily practice, the incidence and morbidity of foot disease in diabetes can be significantly reduced.

Imaging Modalities of the Diabetic Foot 729
Enzo J. Sella and Dawn M. Grosser

Charcot osteoarthropathy is a devastating process that occurs in the diabetic foot. It may be complicated by or confused with osteomyelitis. Osteoarthropathy and osteomyelitis must be differentiated accurately and efficiently because each has different treatments and are potentially limb threatening. This article explores the various available radiologic modalities for distinguishing between the two processes, including plain radiographs, diphosphonate scanning, leukocyte-labeled scans and combined scans, CT, and MR imaging. The combined leukocyte scan with bone marrow imaging is superior to a leukocyte scan alone or in combination with a bone scan for detecting infection in the neuropathic foot. The combined leukocyte scan and marrow imaging is the current gold standard for diagnosis, and MR imaging is the anatomic gold standard to define the extent of the process.

External Fixation in the Management of Charcot Neuroarthropathy **741**
Gary Peter Jolly, Thomas Zgonis, and Vasilios Polyzois

Charcot neuroarthropathy is a complex sequela of neuropathies associated with diabetes mellitus, syringomyelia, alcoholism, and other disorders. The treatment of deformities associated with Charcot neuroarthropathy is evolving from a passive approach to one in which an earlier recognition of the emergence of the event permits an avoidance of deformity. As the understanding of the etiology and natural history of Charcot neuroarthropathy deepens, it has become apparent that many of the deformities that do develop may be reconstructed expeditiously by the surgeon with a thorough understanding of the diabetic foot and experience in the use of external fixation.

Soft Tissue Reconstruction of the Diabetic Foot **757**
Gary Peter Jolly, Thomas Zgonis, and Peter Blume

Treatment of wounds in the diabetic foot presents a set of difficult problems that requires "out of the box" thinking. The traditional approach of off-loading these wounds is often expensive, time-consuming, and in some cases seemingly never ending. The application of the principles and techniques of plastic surgery to the treatment of the foot began in the 1980s, and the integration of these techniques into the armamentarium of the foot and ankle surgeon has progressed quickly. This article will provide an introduction to the principles and methods of soft tissue reconstruction of the diabetic foot.

Elective Surgery of the Diabetic Foot **783**
Lee R. Sayner, Barry I. Rosenblum, and John M. Giurini

Surgical management of the diabetic foot has been limited historically to treatment of ulceration and acute infection. More practitioners now appreciate the role of elective surgery in the treatment and prevention of ulceration, infection, and amputation. This article discusses various elective surgical techniques used to treat the diabetic foot.

Amputation Considerations and Energy Expenditures in the Diabetic Patient **793**
Kathleen Satterfield

Amputations are not procedures of choice but are often necessary and valuable tools for returning a patient who has diabetes to a more active lifestyle. Because of the comorbidities associated with diabetes, this is an important consideration. A return to a more active existence can reduce the effect of vascular disease, hyperglycemic states, and functional limitations. This article addresses the many medical and mobility issues that practitioners should consider before deciding whether to amputate.

Cumulative Index 2003 **803**

Statement of Ownership

Subscription Information

FORTHCOMING ISSUES

January 2004

Arthrodesis Techniques, Part I
Babak Baravarian, DPM, *Guest Editor*

April 2004

Arthrodesis Techniques, Part II
Babak Baravarian, DPM, *Guest Editor*

July 2004

Reconstruction of the Failed Hindfoot, Ankle and Lower Leg Surgery
Walter W. Strash, DPM, *Guest Editor*

RECENT ISSUES

July 2003

Clinical Podogeriatrics: Assessment Education and Prevention
Arthur E. Helfand, DPM, *Guest Editor*

April 2003

Perioperative Management of the Podiatric Patient
Leonard R. Janis, DPM, *Guest Editor*

January 2003

External Fixation of the Foot and Ankle
Jesse B. Burks, DPM, MS, FACFAS, *Guest Editor*

CLINICS IN PODIATRIC MEDICINE AND SURGERY

Clin Podiatr Med Surg
20 (2003) xi–xii

Foreword

Diabetes mellitus

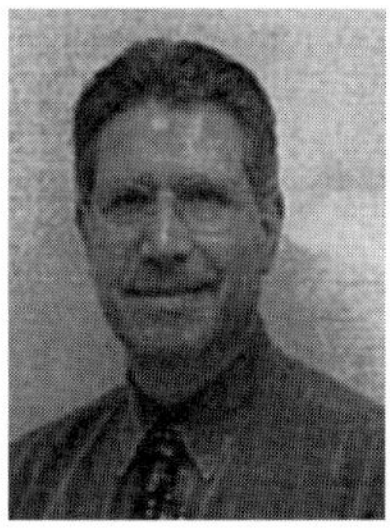

Vincent J. Mandracchia, DPM, MS
Consulting Editor

> Remember that the lowest patient may be your highest hope someday... so treat them accordingly.
>
> —John J. Mollica, MD, 1976

Upon graduating from podiatry school in 1976, I sent a letter to a family physician and good friend of the family and thanked him for his influences and support in my desire to be a physician. Unexpectedly, he sent a letter back, and that one sentence he wrote has affected me more than any other statement regarding my practice goals. I have had the opportunity to teach in two podiatric medical schools and to run a successful practice, and I have reaped the benefits and rewards of both. Today, I work as a full-time, salaried employee of a county hospital, and I see the "lowest" of patients daily: the uninsured, indigent, and less fortunate. On a daily basis I am witness to a lack of commitment to these patients; in fact, often there is a distain for the "inconvenience" of having to treat these patients.

Weekly, we are confronted with an uninsured patient who has been seen in the emergency department of a bigger, more affluent hospital in town and has experienced what is referred to as a "wallet biopsy". Whatever little money the patient has is taken, and they are then referred to a specialist for follow-up—until someone realizes that they are without insurance. They are then told to "go to the county hospital." Why? Besides the obvious EMTALA violations, whatever happened to the oath of the physician? Whatever happened to giving "free care" from time to time as an integral part of a successful practice? Maybe, just maybe, that particular individual who receives free care has a boatload of insured family members. You never know.

0891-8422/03/$ – see front matter
doi:10.1016/S0891-8422(03)00093-4

The ultimate irony at our hospital is the fact that medical students from the allopathic, osteopathic, and podiatric medical institutions in the area clamor for a residency here. This is because of the incredible spectrum of pathology that is experienced in the county system. We train the students and they go on to establish extremely successful and lucrative practices; then, amazingly, they forget their roots and shun any attempt at dispensing free care to the less fortunate. One of the larger hospitals in town touts their institution as the place "where the experts are." We like to think of our hospital as being where the experts *train*.

With success comes the possibility of forgetting that physicians are public servants. After all, without patients we have no practice and subsequently no income. We need to remember that in our dealings with all kinds of patients, and we must be willing to serve those patients with due diligence and skill. I'm often reminded of the words, "There but for the grace of God go I." Scary thought, isn't it?

Drs. Gary Jolly and Thomas Zgonis have tackled a very tough topic in this issue of the *Clinics in Podiatric Medicine and Surgery*: treatment of the diabetic foot. Besides the challenge of dealing with diabetic foot ulcers and Charcot deformities and all the frustrations that accompany them, we need to deal with the whole person, who often is in denial regarding their illness. These patients also have significant comorbidities that complicate their treatment. The expenditure of effort and resources is great, but so are the rewards of preventing amputation and restoring a quality of life for the patient.

Drs. Jolly and Zgonis have compiled a panel of experts in this issue that exemplify a team approach to the complicated diabetic disease entity. This issue is destined to become an excellent reference source for all members of the team that deals with diabetic patients and their associated pedal complications.

Vincent J. Mandracchia, DPM, MS
Broadlawns Medical Center
1801 Hickman Road
Des Moines, IA 50314, USA
E-mail address: vmandracchia@broadlawns.org

CLINICS IN
PODIATRIC
MEDICINE AND
SURGERY

Clin Podiatr Med Surg
20 (2003) xiii–xiv

Preface

Diabetes mellitus

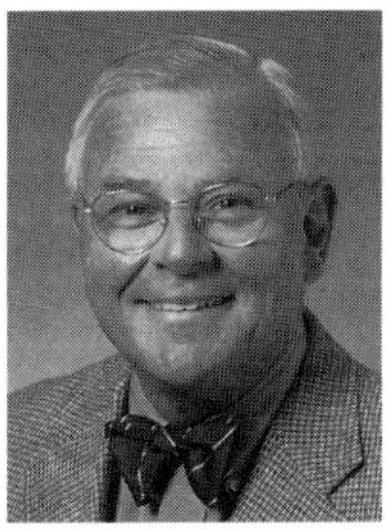

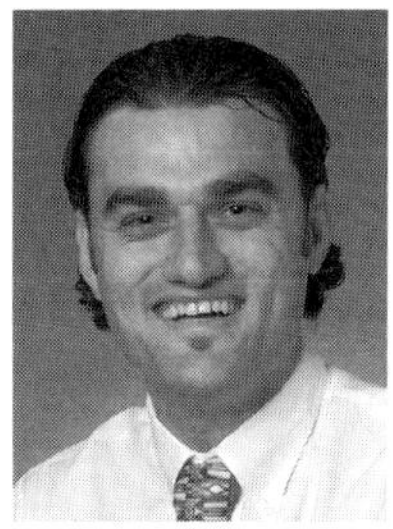

Gary Peter Jolly, DPM, FACFAS   Thomas Zgonis, DPM
Guest Editors

The treatment of the diabetic foot is unquestionably the most difficult thing to do well in the universe of foot and ankle surgery. Patients with ulcers and Charcot deformities require the expenditure of significant resources and often require intensive intervention well after the resolution of their initial problem. Diabetics who develop foot problems rarely do so without developing significant comorbidities, often confusing the pedal diagnosis and making treatment difficult. Peripheral vascular disease, sensory neuropathy, Charcot neuroarthropathy, and histological changes in the skin and connective tissue all contribute to make a bad situation worse.

Advances in the treatment of diabetes, coronary disease, and peripheral vascular disease have resulted in increased life expectancies for patients with these disorders. Because of this, the number of patients presenting with ulcers, lower extremity infections, and Charcot deformities is increasing exponentially. Foot and ankle surgeons are being increasingly challenged by these difficult clinical problems and will require new and more sophisticated solutions to solve them.

The management of the diabetic patient is best done as a team, and should include an internist, an endocrinologist, a vascular surgeon, an infectious disease specialist and a reconstructive foot and ankle surgeon. In addition, diabetic nurse educators and nutritionists play an essential role in aiding these patients manage their disease, and hopefully reduce the risk of diabetic complications. It is in the spirit of the team approach that this issue of the *Clinics in Podiatric Medicine and Surgery* has been written. We are extremely pleased to have been able to bring together this panel of contributing authors, all of whom are extensively published, experts in their individual fields, and actively involved in medical education.

doi:10.1016/S0891-8422(03)00075-2

Their clinical experience and academic accomplishments should be evident from their contributions, which hopefully will be of assistance to the reader.

Gary Peter Jolly, DPM, FACFAS
Thomas Zgonis, DPM
The Center for Reconstructive Foot Surgery
440 New Britain Avenue
Plainville, CT 06062, USA
E-mail addresses: gjolly8060@aol.com (G.P. Jolly)
thomaszgonis@yahoo.com (T. Zgonis)

Clin Podiatr Med Surg
20 (2003) 635–653

CLINICS IN PODIATRIC MEDICINE AND SURGERY

Diabetes mellitus and pharmacological therapy

James Bernene, MD[a], Thomas Zgonis, DPM[b,*], Gary Peter Jolly, DPM, FACFAS[c]

[a]*Department of Medicine, New Britain General Hospital, New Britain, CT 06052, USA*
[b]*The Center for Reconstructive Foot Surgery, 440 New Britain Avenue, Plainville, CT 06062, USA*
[c]*Department of Podiatric Surgery, New Britain General Hospital, New Britain, CT 06052, USA*

Diabetes ("running through") mellitus ("honeyed") was first defined in ancient Rome in the first century AD. The Roman physician Aretaeus attributed the disease to a large amount of sugar in the urine that led in to a coma and eventual death within weeks or months. Patients would taste their own urine to diagnose high blood sugar levels in their bodies [1]. Today, diabetes mellitus (DM) has been defined as a group of metabolic disorders in which there is impaired glucose use, which have in common chronic hyperglycemia [2]. Diabetes mellitus has also been defined as a chronic disorder affecting carbohydrate, fat, and protein metabolism that is caused by lack or insufficient use of insulin in the body [3].

Chronic hyperglycemia, along with other metabolic abnormalities associated with diabetes, has been shown to increase the risk of heart disease, kidney failure, retinopathy nerve damage, and amputations. The metabolic, vascular, and neuropathic components of the disease need to be addressed closely to avoid major complications, including death [3].

Incidence

In the United States there are approximately 17 million people with diabetes, of whom about 6 million people are undiagnosed. Some 625,000 new cases are seen annually. The disease is more prevalent in Hispanic/Latino community, non-Hispanic blacks, and Native Americans. Between 90% and 95% of the diagnosed diabetics are type 2, and 5% and 10% are type 1. Diabetes mellitus (DM) is the seventh leading cause of death and the number one cause of atraumatic amputations, end-stage renal disease, and blindness in the United States [4].

* Corresponding author.
E-mail address: thomaszgonis@yahoo.com (T. Zgonis).

doi:10.1016/S0891-8422(03)00066-1

Classification, diagnosis, and screening

The old classification in 1979 by the National Diabetes Data Group (NDDG) was updated in 1997 by the American Diabetes Association (ADA). The old classification categorized the diabetic patients into two groups: type I (IDDM) and type II (NIDDM). Table 1 shows the two major classifications made in 1979 [5,6].

The classification system by the NDDG in 1979 added other categories in addition to the changes listed in Table 1. Gestational diabetes and other conditions and syndromes associated with diabetes and impaired glucose tolerance became a subclass of diabetes mellitus. Fasting plasma glucose was set at greater than or equal to 140 mg/dl on more than one occasion, and the Oral Glucose Tolerance Test (OGTT) was set at greater than or equal to 200 mg/dl between 0 and 2 hours. The OGTT was standardized to 75 g carbohydrate dose in nonpregnant adults [5].

In 1997, ADA added and clarified the following classifications:

Type 1 DM (beta cell destruction leading to lack of insulin) and type 2 DM (progressive insulin secretory defect in a background of insulin resistance) instead of IDDm and NIDDM

Gestational diabetes mellitus (GDM), diagnosed during pregnancy

Other types of diabetes mellitus; genetic defects on beta cell function, chemical or drug induced; diseases of the exocrine pancreas; infections; and genetic defects in insulin action

Individuals with transient hyperglycemia due to spontaneous stimuli or those with abnormal glucose tolerance who are unable to meet the diagnostic criteria for DM can be considered to have impaired fasting glucose or impaired glucose tolerance [7,8].

Table 1
NDDG classification in 1979

Type I/IDDM (10–20%)	Type II/NIDDM (80–90%)
Onset <20 years old; normal weight; decreased blood insulin	Onset >30 years old; normal or increased blood insulin
Juvenile onset diabetes	Insulin resistance
Islet cell antibodies	No islet cell antibodies
Ketoacidosis is common	Ketoacidosis is rare
50% concordance in twins; HLA-D linked	90–100% concordance in twins; no HLA-D association
Autoimmunity; severe insulin deficiency	Relative insulin deficiency
Early insulitis	No insulitis
Beta cell depletion; must receive insulin to control diabetes	Mild beta cell depletion
Marked atrophy and fibrosis of islet cells	Focal atrophy and amyloid islet cells

The newest criteria for diagnosing DM include the following:

Symptoms of diabetes (polyuria, polyphagia, polydipsia, and unexplained weight loss) and random plasma glucose greater or equal to 200mg/dl;
Fasting plasma glucose (no caloric intake for at least 8 hours) greater or equal to 126 mg/dl; or
A glucose level of 200 mg/dl or greater during an Oral Glucose Tolerance Test (OGTT) between 0 and 2 hours

Screening for DM should start at age 45 and be repeated every 3 years in individuals without risk factors, and earlier and more often for those with risk factors. Risk factors include relatives with diabetes, obesity, certain ethnic groups, hypertension, history of gestational diabetes, and increased lipid profiles. In addition, testing for type 2 diabetes in children should be performed in those who have a mean body mass index above the 95th percentile and a positive family history, certain ethnicities, a sedentary lifestyle, or conditions associated with insulin resistance (HTN, dyslipidemia, and acanthosis nigricans). These children should be tested every 2 years starting at the age of 10 years [7–13].

Normal insulin metabolism and glucose homeostasis

Insulin is a hormone secreted by the beta cells in the pancreas. The function of insulin is to maintain a glucose homeostasis through two principle mechanisms: (1) stimulation of glucose uptake by muscle and fat tissue and (2) suppression of hepatic glucose production and fat breakdown, thereby inhibiting free fatty acid release

Blood glucose is under tight control (60–140 mg/dl) in nondiabetics. This is accomplished by interplay between insulin and all the anti-insulins (glucagon, cortisol, catecholamines, and growth hormone) and their regulation of glucose production and disposal. Hyperglycemia secondary to impaired or absent insulin in the body contributes to the development of chronic vascular complications and needs to be addressed aggressively once it is diagnosed [2].

Pathogenesis of type 1 diabetes mellitus

Type 1 DM is a lifelong disease and is characterized by a severe, absolute lack of insulin caused by a destruction of the pancreatic beta cells. It develops most commonly early in life, and patients depend on exogenous insulin for survival. It can occur at any age in life, however, depending on the severity of the disease. Sudden onset and ketoacidosis, which often leads to the diagnosis, are common in these individuals. Patients newly diagnosed with type 1 diabetes often have a transient return to normal glucose homeostasis for 6 to 12 months (the "honeymoon phase") before a more permanent beta cell failure and hyperglycemia ensue [14].

The pathogenesis of type 1 DM can be attributed to two major factors responsible for the islet beta cell destruction: genetic susceptibility and environmental influence. The major genetic susceptibility is most commonly associated with HLA-DR3 and HLA-DR4. The presence of histocompatibility antigens, such as B8 and B15, are also strongly associated with type 1 DM [14–18]. Environmental factors that can lead to destruction of beta cells include viruses such as cocksackie B, mumps, measles, and cytomegalovirus [19–21]. Bacterial infections in Caucasians with a higher percentage of islet cell antibodies increase the risk of developing type 1 diabetes. Cow's milk ingestion in early life (not being breast-fed beyond the age of 3 months) was thought to also increase the risk of type 1 DM [2,22–24]. This is controversial, however, and a recent study by Hummel et al [25] showed no evidence of environmental factors affecting islet antibody in the first 2 years of life in offspring of parents with type 1 diabetes.

Associations with other autoimmune diseases including Grave's, Addison's, and Hashimoto's thyroiditis are common, and islet cell antibodies may be found in each of these conditions. Most common autoantibodies found in type 1 diabetics include the islet cell autoantibodies (ICA), autoantibodies to insulin (IAA), autoantibodies to tyrosinephosphatases (IA-2), and autoantibodies to glutamic decarboxylase (GAD65) [26,27]. All of these serve as markers for the disease and tests for them are available in most commercial laboratories.

Pathogenesis of type 2 diabetes mellitus

Type 2 DM is characterized by two metabolic defects: relative or absolute insulin deficiency or inability of peripheral tissues to respond to insulin (insulin resistance). Impaired insulin secretion and insulin resistance may be seen individually or in combination. Insulin resistance by peripheral tissues requires the pancreas to produce more insulin to maintain normal glucose homeostasis. Overproduction of glucose by the liver and inadequate glucose uptake by muscle overwhelms the pancreas's ability to produce insulin and results in progressively higher blood sugar levels.

Insulin resistance is associated with obesity in the vast majority of type 2 patients. Although the mechanism for this is incompletely understood, free fatty acids probably play an important role in the insulin resistance syndrome. The association between obesity, hypertension, and dyslipidemia is well established and accounts for the high incidence of macrovascular disease in these patients [28].

Signs and symptoms of diabetes mellitus

Acute symptoms of DM include frequent urination, increased thirst and hunger, unexplained weight loss, fatigue, and mental changes. Symptoms develop quickly in patients with type 1 diabetes and more slowly, often over several months or years, in patients with type 2 diabetes. Symptoms might be first noticed after an acute illness or during a routine medical visit. It is estimated that currently some 8 million people have DM but are undiagnosed. Vascular complications, including the heart and large blood vessels, kidney, and eye disease, nonhealing wounds, hypertension, and obesity, are some of the factors that are associated with DM [28,29].

Hyperglycemia is the hallmark of the disease and can lead to glycosuria, which occurs when the plasma glucose exceeds the renal threshold for glucose reabsorption (180 mg/dl). This osmotic diuresis causes water to be drawn into the urine with the glucose, resulting in polyuria. Polyuria leads to dehydration, hyperosmolality, electrolyte imbalance, increased thirst, and thus polydipsia. Polyphagia results from the significant loss of glucose into the urine. For each gram of urinary glucose there is a 4.5 calorie per day loss that produces a compensatory increase in food intake in an attempt to balance the daily loss of glucose.

Other acute signs and symptoms include generalized weakness, fatigue, transient visual blurring, frequent urinary tract infections, candida vaginitis, thrush, and pruritus. Late complications of diabetes include diabetic microangiopathy (diffuse thickening of basement membranes in skeletal muscles, retina, placenta, and renal glomeruli), atherosclerosis (myocardial infarction, gangrene of the lower extremities, and cerebral vascular accidents), diabetic retinopathy (vitreous hemorrhages and retinal detachments), diabetic nephropathy (hypertension, papillitis, glomerulosclerosis, and urinary tract infections), and diabetic neuropathy (symmetric bilateral peripheral neuropathy and autonomic dysfunction—gastroparesis, postural hypotension, neurogenic bladder, and impotence).

Diabetic ketoacidosis (DKA) is most commonly found in patients with type 1 DM and is usually precipitated by an infection, resulting in severe insulin deficiency coupled with absolute or relative increase of glucagon production. Insulin depletion triggers lipolysis as an alternative source for the production of glucose, which results in the production of free fatty acids (FFA). FFA are oxidized into ketone bodies in the liver, which leads to ketonemia, ketonuria, and metabolic ketoacidosis that may eventually lead to encephalopathy, cardiac arrhythmias, and death. Nonketotic hyperosmolar syndrome is found usually in elderly patients with type 2 diabetes who become severely volume depleted, confused, and thus unable to seek medical care. Volume depletion secondary to severe dehydration may also lead to a diabetic coma [29,30].

Laboratory evaluation of patients admitted in diabetic coma should include frequent testing of blood sugar levels, arterial blood gases, serum electrolyte, and creatinine levels; urinalysis for ketones and protein;, a careful search for infection; and cardiac monitoring. Rapid treatment with intravenous fluids and insulin is mandatory [14].

Oral hypoglycemic drugs

Oral hypoglycemic agents are generally indicated in patients with type 2 DM only. Patients most commonly start pharmacological therapy when diet, exercise, and other life modifications are not enough to control their blood sugars. Type 2 patients are typically started on a single agent and their blood sugars are mentioned for 2 to 3 months. At the end of that time a second and sometimes a third agent may be introduced. The goal of therapy is to maintain hemoglobin A1C levels less than 6.5% to 7%.

The following seven classes of oral hypoglycemic agents are currently used in the United States:

Sulfonylureas (first and second generation)
Biguanides (Glucophage)
Thiazolidinediones/TZDs (Avandia, Actos, Rezulin)
Alpha-glucosidase inhibitors (Glyset, Precose)
Meglitinides (Prandin, Starlix)
Combinations (Glucovance, Avandamet, Metaglip)

Sulfonylureas

The sulfonylureas are the oldest oral hypoglycemics and were first developed during World War II. It was discovered that in certain patients, sulfonamide use had detrimental hypoglycemic effects. The first sulfonylurea agent was used in Germany in 1955 (Carbutamide). The original first-generation sulfonylureas include all the agents developed from 1950s to the 1970s. The second-generation sulfonylureas include all the agents developed from the 1980s and thereafter (Tables 2 and 3). The second-generation agents have essentially replaced the first-generation drugs because of their longer duration with less frequent dosing and fewer side effects [31].

Sulfonylureas stimulate pancreatic beta cells to secrete insulin. These agents are only effective in patients with functioning islet cells. Their mechanisms of action include closing the potassium channels in pancreatic beta cell membranes and depolarization, which triggers insulin release. The most common side effects include hypoglycemia, weight gain, sulfa allergy, and the production of a metallic taste. Potential risk for adverse effects on the liver and the introduction of several other newer classes of drugs have decreased the popularity of these agents [32,33]. These drugs have reported interactions with sulfonamides, chloramphenicol, phenylbutazone, propranolol, and ethanol. Drinking alcohol with these medica-

Table 2
First generation sulfonylurea agents

Brand name (generic)	Daily dose (mg)	Metab/excretion	Duration of action (h)
Orinase (tolbutamide)	500–2500	Liver	6–12
Diabinese (chlorpropamide)	100–500	Kidney	60
Tolinase (tolazamide)	100–1000	Liver	12–24
Dymelor (acetohexamide)	250–1500	Liver/kidney	12–18

Table 3
Second generation sulfonylurea agents

Brand name (generic)	Daily dose (mg)	Metab/excretion	Duration of action (h)
Micronase/Diabeta (glyburide)	1.5–20	Liver/kidney	12–24
Glucotrol/Glucotrol XL (glipizide)	5–20	Liver/kidney	12–24
Amaryl (glimepiride)	1–8	Liver/kidney	16–24

tions can cause heart palpitations and flushing. Physicians should be aware of all sulfa-containing drugs when sulfonylurea pharmacotherapy is initiated [34–37].

Biguanides

Metformin (Glucophage) is the only biguanide available in the United States. Metformin and phenformin were developed in the mid-1950s; however, phenformin was withdrawn from the US market because of a significant risk of severe lactic acidosis [38,39]. Metformin has been in the US market since 1994 with fewer side effects and promising outcomes. Metformin is also used in combined oral hypoglycemic agents.

Biguanides reduce the rate of gluconeogenesis in the liver. They also stimulate glycolysis in the peripheral tissues, which increases insulin sensitivity and reduces the production of glucagon. Biguanides also act by reducing the absorption of glucose from the gut.

The main targeting organ of metformin is the liver, with secondary effects on muscle and fat. The duration of action is 8 hours and the time to reach maximum effect varies from 2 to 4 hours. Metformin as monotherapy has been found to lower Hgb A1C by 1.5% 2%. The dose can range between 500 and 2500 mg/day. Glucophage XR, a sustained release form, is available and taken only once a day. Side effects include abdominal discomfort with diarrhea and bloating, a metallic taste, and, rarely, lactic acidosis (1/33,000 years of use). This is almost always seen in patients with some form of renal insufficiency.

Metformin has been shown to have virtually no risk of causing hypoglycemia, and patients taking metformin have been found to experience mild weight reduction and improved lipid levels by reducing triglycerides and LDL cholesterol and increasing HDL cholesterol. Metformin may be used with insulin to lessen insulin requirements in patients with type 2 diabetes who are taking insulin. Combination therapy with sulfonylureas leads to a further reduction of blood sugars and Hgb A1C levels.

As noted previously, lactic acidosis has been associated with biguanides. It is seen most commonly in patients with renal insufficiency and older individuals. Metformin is contraindicated in patients with kidney or liver disease and should be used with caution in patients with congestive heart failure or a history of a diabetic ketoacidosis. Lactic acidosis can be also triggered by the consumption of alcohol in patients taking metformin, and so this drug should be avoided in patients with a history of alcohol abuse. Finally, metformin is witheld following any procedure with an intravenous dye, such as angiograms, CT scans, and intravenous pyelograms. Intravenous radio-opaque dyes can trigger transient acute renal failure and lead to lactic acidosis in patients taking metformin. The drug should be withheld the day of the procedure and for at least 48 hours following the procedure or until the serum creatinine has returned to baseline [40–43].

Thiazolidinediones (TZDs)

The only TZDs or glitazones available in the United States are rosiglitazone (Avandia) and pioglitazone (Actos). Troglitazone (Rezulin) was the first glitazone released but was withdrawn from the market because of severe hepatotoxicity and a number of deaths [44,45]. Glitazones have few advantages over sulfonylureas or metformin as monotherapy, but in combination with these agents have been shown to improve glycemic control [46]. Glitazones are designed to improved insulin sensitivity in muscle, liver, and fat cells and are often referred to as insulin-sensitizing agents.

Glitazones work by reversing insulin resistance and improving insulin sensitivity in the liver and in peripheral tissues. Glitazones exert their major metabolic effect through activation of the peroxisome proliferator activated receptor gamma (PPAR-gamma). PPAR-gammas are transcription factors that regulate the expression of numerous genes influencing carbohydrate and lipid metabolism. Glitazones decrease hepatic glucose production, reduce free fatty acid concentration, improve beta cell function, and may prolong beta cell survival.

Glitazones have duration of action of about 8 hours and reach maximum effect in 2 to 4 hours. They typically lower HgA1C by 1% to 1.5%. The dose range varies from 15 to 45 mg/d for pioglitazone and 2 to 8 mg/d for rosiglitazone. Side effects of these drugs include headache, diarrhea, muscle weakness, fatigue, and fluid retention.

These agents have their greatest effect on the blood sugar immediately after eating and should be taken with meals. Monotherapy with the glitazones rarely causes hypoglycemia, but if used with sulfonylureas or insulin the risk increases significantly [47,48].

Glitazones have also been found to lower free fatty acids and triglycerides while increasing plasma HDL levels. They are associated with a fairly low incidence of liver abnormalities, but monitoring liver function before starting treatment, and every 2 months for the first year of treatment, is highly recommended. The drug should be stopped if Alanine Aminotransaminase/Aspartate Aminotransaminase (ALT/AST) are found to be significantly elevated (threefold) after the treatment is initiated.

Glitazones are effective in the treatment of type 2 diabetes caused by insulin resistance. One side effect associated with glitazones—fluid retention—may aggravate underlying congestive heart failure and is therefore contraindicated in such patients. These drugs can be effectively combined with sulfonylureas, metformin, or insulin for better glycemic levels and reduction of Hgb A1C.

Alpha glucosidase inhibitors

The two agents in this group include acarbose (Precose) and miglitol (Glycet). These drugs are different from those in the other groups in that they work by decreasing the production of glucose from carbohydrates in the gut. If glucose levels rise slowly after meals, endogenous insulin can respond more effectively than if there is a rapid rise. Acarbose was first introduced in the United States in 1996, and miglitol was recently approved by the FDA for use in this country [49].

The mechanism of action of alpha glucosidase inhibitors is based on the inhibition of the production of alpha glucosidase enzymes in the small intestine. These proteins are involved in starch degradation in the gut. The alpha glucosidase inhibitors also act by inhibiting the secretion of sucrase, inhibiting the absorption of monosaccharides.

The main target organ of acarbose and miglitol is the small intestine. The duration of action of these drugs is 4 hours and the time to reach maximum effect is about 1 hour. It has been shown to lower Hgb A1C by 0.5% to 1%. The dose range varies from 12.5 to 100 mg before each meal. Common side effects associated with these drugs include abdominal pain, nausea, diarrhea, and bloating and are limiting factors in their use.

Monotherapy with the alpha glucosidase inhibitors does not cause hypoglycemia or weight gain. They can be added to other oral hypoglycemics for better glycemic levels and are a good choice for either type 1 or type 2 diabetics. There is a low incidence of systemic toxicity, but their use in type 1 diabetics is not FDA approved.

The major disadvantage to the use of these agents is the gastrointestinal side effects. Many patients experience significant abdominal pain, diarrhea, bloating, and flatulence. These effects can sometimes be prevented by starting the patient on lower doses initially and slightly increasing the dose over a period of 2 to 4 months. Alpha glucosidase inhibitors are contraindicated in individuals with inflammatory bowel disease or liver disease [50,51].

Meglitinides

The two agents in this group include repaglinide (Prandin) and nateglinide (Starlix). These drugs are sulfonylurea-like agents and increase pancreatic insulin and release by a different mechanism. They are also known as insulin secretagogues and prandial glucose regulators. Hypoglycemia is less frequent with these drugs than with the sulfonylurea drugs because of their shorter duration and more rapid peak of action. They are the newest oral hypoglycemics for the treatment of type 2 DM [52,53].

Meglitinides require the presence of glucose to close the ATP-sensitive potassium sensitive channels and induce calcium influx, which stimulates endogenous insulin secretion. This mechanism is most important in first-phase insulin secretion and rapidly turns off as blood glucose begins to fall in the late postprandial period.

The main targeting organ of the meglitinides is the beta cell with a duration of action of 3 hours, reaching a maximum effect at 1 hour. Repaglinide and nateglinide have been shown to lower Hgb A1c levels by 0.5% to 0.7%. Dosing ranges vary from 0.5 to 4 mg before each meal for repaglinide and 60 to120 mg before each meal for nateglinide. Side effects from these drugs are rare but include hypoglycemia, nausea and vomiting, diarrhea, headache, and muscle and joint aches.

For meglitinides to be effective, the patient must have functional beta cells present, and so are ineffective in patients with type 1 DM. They are ideally taken 10 to 30 minutes before each meal. The risk for hypoglycemia in patients taking repaglinide or nateglinide is low because they are quickly absorbed and rapidly eliminated by the biliary system. For this reason, meglitinides should not be used in patients with liver disease. However, they can be used safely in patients with renal insufficiency. It has been shown to have a synergistic effect with metformin in reducing Hgb A1C levels. Meglitinides have demonstrated drug interactions with sulfonamides, probenecid, NSAIDS, calcium channel blockers, thiazide diuretics, and corticosteroids and should be used with caution in patients taking these agents [54].

Oral combination pharmacotherapy

The three agents in this group include metformin HCL/glyburide (Glucovance), rosiglitazone maleate/metformin HCL (Avandamet), and glipizide/metformin HCL (Metaglip).

Metformin HCL/glyburide contains biguanide and sulfonyurea agents and lowers the blood sugar by stimulating the beta cell to release more insulin and inhibiting hepatic gluconeogenesis. The combination causes a greater decrease in blood sugars and Hgb A1c levels than metformin or glyburide alone. Dosages range from 250/1.25 to 2000/20 mg daily. The same precautions should be taken for the biguanides and sulfonylureas if they were being used alone [39].

Rosiglitazone maleate/metformin HCL contains a glitazone and a biguanide and dosages include 1/500, 2/500, and 4/500 mg twice a day. This combination drug causes a more significant change in blood sugar than either a glitazone or biguanide alone [55].

Glipizide/metformin HCL contains a biguanide and a sulfonylurea agent similar to that of metformin HCL/glyburide. Dosages range from 2.5/250 mg/day in initial therapy to 5/500 mg twice a day. The same precautions and warnings should be taken as with all the sulfonylureas and biguanides. Lactic acidosis is a rare but serious condition resulting from metformin accumulation [56].

Insulin therapy

Insulin is secreted by the beta cells of the pancreas and facilitates cellular absorption of glucose and the maintenance of a normal glucose homeostasis.

Patients with type 1 DM, whose beta cells are depleted or destroyed, depend entirely on exogenous insulin for the rest of their lives. Insulin is also prescribed in individuals with type 2 DM when exercise, diet, and oral hypoglycemics are inadequate to maintain normal glucose levels, which is usually later in the course of the disease and when endogenous insulin secretion begins to fail. Exogenous insulin is also used in pregnancy in women with gestational diabetes when oral hypoglycemics are contraindicated [57].

Exogenous insulin comes from two sources: animals and genetically engineered bacteria. The latter produces an insulin that is similar to that of human insulin. Exogenous insulins replace endogenous insulin and have all the effects of endogenous insulin by decreasing hepatic gluconeogenesis and enhancing glucose uptake by the peripheral tissues. Their uses tend to promote weight gain, risk of hyperinsulinemia, and hypoglycemia. Insulin therapy can be used for a short term, such as during perioperative periods, or as a definitive therapy [58].

The different types of insulins are categorized according to their onset, peak time, and duration of action. Insulins may be thought of as rapid acting, short acting, intermediate acting, and long acting. Insulins may be found in mixture to make administration easier for the patient. The route of administration is usually subcutaneously (SQ), but certain insulins can be given intravenously (IV) in patients who are ill or preoperatively. Various routes of administration can be used, including insulin pens, insulin pumps, or inhaled or oral insulin. The classes of insulin with their onset, peak, and duration of action are shown in Table 4.

The rapid-acting insulins include the human insulins lispro (Humalog) and aspart (Novolog). Lispro was the first designer insulin to be approved in the United States in 1996; aspart was approved in 2001. Lispro is produced by recombinant DNA technology in vitro by reversing the amino acid sequence in the 28th and 29th position in the beta chain and switching lysine and proline, hence the name lispro. Aspart is produced by a similar process, but the substitution is aspartic acid for proline. Both rapid-acting insulins are quickly absorbed in the bloodstream, peak

Table 4
Insulin regimes available in the United States

Insulin	Preparation	Onset	Peak	Duration (h)
Rapid acting	Humalog (Lispro)[a]	5–15 min	30–90 min	3–5
	Novolog (Aspart)[a]	5–15 min	40–50 min	3–5
Short acting	Regular (CZI)[a]	30–60 min	2–4 h	4–6
Intermediate acting	NPH	2–4	6–10 h	14–16
	Lente	3–4	6–12 h	16–18
	75/25 (NPL/lispro)	15–60 min	1–6½ h	10–16
	70/30 (NPH/regular)	30–60 min	2–10 h	10–16
	50/50 (NPH/regular)	30–60 min	1–10 h	10–16
Long acting	Ultralente	4–6 h	8–18 h	18–24
	Lantus[a]	2–3 h	No peak	18–26

Abbreviations: NPH, neutral protamine hagedorn; NPL, neutral protamine lispro; CZI, crystalline zinc insulin.

[a] Indicates all the clear insulins.

less than 30 minutes after injection, and last only for 3 to 4 hours. Their great advantage is that they are associated with a smaller rise in blood glucose after meals and lesser risk of postabsorptive hypoglycemia. Studies have shown that they are equally effective and provided similar pump compatibility with regular insulin when used in continuous subcutaneous insulin infusion. The dose should be given at the time of the meal or up to 10 minutes before. These rapid-acting insulins should be used in combination with intermediate- and long-acting insulins [59–66].

Regular insulin is the only insulin approved in the United States labeled as short acting. It was first made available in 1922. The onset of regular insulin is 30 minutes; it peaks at about 3 to 4 hours and has a total duration of action of about 6 to 8 hours. Regular insulin is produced by recombinant DNA technology in vitro. Patients usually inject regular insulin 30 minutes before their meals. Regular insulin is a clear, colorless solution and is usually less expensive than the rapid-acting insulins. Regular insulin is preferred for emergency cases with profound hyperglycemia because of its longer duration than that of rapid-acting insulins [57].

Intermediate-acting insulins include NPH, Lente, and all the premixed insulins. NPH (human insulin rDNA isophane suspension) is produced by a genetically engineered strain of *E coli*. It is a crystalline suspension with protamine and zinc. The function of protamine in NPH (30–50 mg/100U) is to delay the absorption of insulin. NPH is used subcutaneously only and cannot be given intravenously. It has a slow onset of action and may last up to 16 hours. Side effects include hypoglycemia and, rarely, lipodystrophy. Lente insulin is a mixture of 30% Semilente and 70% Ultralente insulins. Lente insulin should not be mixed with NPH or regular insulin because it can delay the onset of the short-acting insulin. Lente's duration is slightly longer than that of NPH and like NPH is only given subqutaneously. Premixed insulins (NPH/regular or lispro mixtures) come in several different forms, including 70/30, 75/25, and 50/50, and offer the patient greater flexibility in dosing. Combination therapy of premixed insulin and oral hypoglycemics has shown promise in treating type 2 patients who require insulin [67].

Long-acting insulins include Ultralente and Glargine. Ultralente (extended insulin zinc suspension) is a cloudy insulin and was the only long-acting insulin available in the United States. Total duration of action is up to 24 hours. Glargine (Lantus) is a recombinant DNA human insulin analoq genetically engineered from *E coli*. It is a clear insulin and cannot be mixed with any other insulin. Its duration is between 18 and 26 hours and can be given once a day, normally at bedtime. The use of long-acting insulins provides a basal insulin level that is fairly constant in the fasting or premeal time periods [68–70].

Innovations in insulin therapy

Intermediate- or long-acting insulin at bedtime either alone or in combination with oral hypoglycemic agents has been proposed in recent years for the treatment of type 2 diabetes. Bedtime insulin suppresses nocturnal gluconeogenesis and is less likely to produce hypoglycemic episodes. Combination therapy of bedtime insulin and oral hypoglycemics also minimizes the risk of weight gain and may reduce the insulin dose by 50% to 60% when compared with multiple daily insulin injection regimens [60].

There are three commonly used insulin regimens. The first consists of one injection per day with an intermediate- or long-acting insulin given at night and an oral agent(s) during the day. A second protocol involves two injections per day containing a rapid- or short-acting insulin and an intermediate-acting one. Either of these two protocols can be used in type 2 patients. For patients with type 1 diabetes, three injections or more per day have been advocated consisting of a rapid- or short-acting insulin combined with a long-acting insulin at bedtime. Therefore, a combination of intermediate- and short- or rapid-acting insulin before breakfast and supper works better for patients with type 2 diabetes, whereas a combination of rapid or short acting before each meal and long acting at bedtime works better for patients with type 1 diabetes. The rapid- or short-acting insulin provides a high level of insulin during glucose absorption from the intestine and the long-acting insulin provides a low level of insulin needed during fasting hours [58,71–78].

Glucose monitoring

For patients with type 1 diabetes, blood sugar levels should be tested at least four times a day (before breakfast, lunch, supper, and at bedtime) and adjustments should be made accordingly. Hemoglobin A1c (glycosylated hemoglobin) is a time-integrated measure of the prevailing glucose concentration to which red blood cells have been exposed and indicates the average blood sugar levels for the preceding 3 to 4 months. Hgb A1c levels should be used as a basis for adjusting insulin therapy and should provide the physician with a reasonably good idea of the patient's glycemic levels over a long period of time. Studies have been shown that a 1% reduction in Hgb A1c levels reduces the risk of diabetes-related deaths by 21% [79]. Therefore, it should be the goal of the patient and the physician to maintain Hgb A1c levels below 6.5% to 7% (125–140 mg/dl blood glucose).

Perioperative management of diabetes mellitus

Surgery on diabetic patients should usually be performed early in the morning, and in elective cases only after glycemic control can be established. Patients who have diabetes have a longer hospital stay than patients without diabetes because of their multiple organ pathologies superimposed on their surgical procedures. More than 50% of all nontraumatic lower extremity amputations in the United States occur in individuals with DM. The quality of inpatient management of DM in American hospitals has been shown to be suboptimal. Diabetes mellitus is not considered as a primary diagnosis and is often not treated aggressively in the inpatient setting, particularly when diabetic patients are admitted to surgical services. Vascular, cardiopulmonary, and renal diseases are given greater attention with an aggressive approach to prophylaxis, and relegating the management of DM often takes a back seat [80].

Surgeons should be aware of the detrimental effects of elevated blood sugars before, during, and after any surgical procedure. Wound healing is affecting by hyperglycemia. Diabetic patients who are poorly controlled have significantly higher risk of infection, impairing skin fibroblast activity and impaired growth factor function. Diabetic patients are also prone to dehydration, fluid overload, and electrolyte imbalance during the perioperative period. In addition, abnormal platelet aggregation is seen in diabetics, and excessive bleeding or accelerated clotting can occur. Most diabetics who present with neuropathy and subsequent ulceration also demonstrate poor nutrition as evidenced by abnormally low serum albumins [80–86].

Type 2 diabetic patients

In the patient with well-controlled type 2 diabetes, oral hypoglycemics should be discontinued before surgery and given only when the patient has resumed eating postoperatively. Metformin should be withheld until at least 48 hours after surgery because of a possible perioperative alteration in renal function affecting metformin levels. In patients being treated with oral hypoglycemic agents and insulin, the oral hypoglycemics and the rapid- or short-acting insulin should be held before surgery. There is some disagreement about how much intermediate- or long-acting insulin should be administered. Dosages vary from 50% to 100%. Sole sliding scales should be avoided because they only offer a fluctuating glycemic control. Greater reliance on insulin infusions in the immediate post-operative period should be the rule with meticulous control of blood sugar (120–140 mg/dl).

Anesthesia regulations require the patients not to eat or drink for 12 hours before surgery. If surgery is scheduled early in the morning, the above criteria should be followed with the addition of intravenous fluids, such as lactated Ringer's solution or normal saline. However, if surgery is to be performed later in the day, the same regimen should be followed with the substitution of D5W1/2NS as intravenous fluids during the morning of surgery. The rate of infusion should be adjusted to the patient's renal function and cardiac considerations. Sliding scale can then be used for glycemic control, but only until the first postoperative day.

An excellent alternative regimen is to begin an insulin/glucose infusion with D5W1/2NS and piggyback insulin drip with 100U in 201 cc 0.5 NS to deliver 0.5 to 2 U/h. This regimen requires hourly capillary blood sugar measurements for adjustment to keep blood sugar between 100 and 150 mg/dl. Finger sticks to test blood sugars are also important before, during, and after the surgical procedure to provide better control of blood sugars.

Type 1 diabetic patients

Patients with type 1 diabetes rely on exogenous insulin, but their perioperative management should be almost the same as the type 2 diabetic patient. Rapid- or short-acting insulin should be on hold the day of surgery and one half or two thirds of the morning or bedtime long-acting insulin should be administered. If the patient goes to surgery later in the day, hydration with D5W 0.5 NSS should be started at 75 to 125 cc/h the morning of surgery. If surgery is performed early in the morning, hydration with lactated Ringer's solution is also acceptable.

An alternative to the above regimen is to place the patient on an insulin drip as described above [80,82,86]. Blood sugar monitoring before, during, and after surgery are important, and necessary treatments should be initiated with small doses of rapid- or short-acting insulin.

Goals for normal glucose levels

The physician should be aware of the treatment for hypoglycemia, the other extreme, during the perioperative period. To minimize the risk of hypoglycemia, blood sugars should be slightly higher at bedtime and before breakfast. Patients with diabetes also need to be monitored by the nursing staff for potential hypoglycemia. Although some patients know when they become hypoglycemic, others do not and require closer supervision. Hypertension is extremely common in diabetics and treatment involves the use of a variety of antihypertensive agents. Common antihypertensive drugs include angiotensin-converting enzyme (ACE) inhibitors and angiotensin II receptor-blockers. ACE inhibitors have also been proven to decrease the risk of progression of nephropathy and cardiovascular events in type 1 and type 2 patients, respectively. Beta blockers are useful in diabetics for their cardio-protective effects but should be used with caution in all diabetics and particularly those prone to hypoglycemic effects. They not only inhibit the adrenergic symptoms (diaphoresis, palpitations) but also inhibit catecholamine-stimulated gluconeogenesis [87].

Treatment of hypoglycemia

Symptoms of hypoglycemia include sweating, tremor, palpitations, and irritability. Severe hypoglycemia can cause convulsions and unresponsiveness. Hypoglycemia needs to be treated immediately to avoid any major systemic complications. For mild hypoglycemia, 10 to 20 g of oral glucose or a glass of orange juice is probably adequate to raise the blood sugar to normal levels. For severe hypoglycemia, intravenous D5W (0.5–1 g/kg) or glucagon (1 mg) IM as a one-time dose should be administered until normal blood sugar levels are established. Blood sugars should be monitored every 1 to 2 hours until normal values are achieved especially if the hypoglycemia is the result of a longer-acting sulfonylurea or insulin preparation [88,89].

Summary

Diabetes mellitus can be a devastating lifelong disease if not treated appropriately. The physician and the patient should be aware of both extremes involved with DM: hyperglycemia and hypoglycemia. Patient education and preventive care are perhaps more important in this disease than many others. A multidisciplinary approach involving the patient, physician, and diabetic educator is best to assure a better quality of life. Enormous advances in the treatment of diabetes have occurred over the past decade and even greater ones can be expected in the future. New drugs, insulin delivery devices, and noninvasive glucose monitoring machines have the potential to normalize blood sugar levels and return diabetics to a near normal lifespan without complications [90,91].

References

[1] Marble A. Correct concepts of diabetes. In: Joslin's diabetes mellitus. 11th edition. Philadelphia: Lea & Febiger; 1971. p. 884.
[2] Robbins SL. Diabetes mellitus. In: Cotran R, Kumar V, Robbins S, editors. Robbins pathologic basis of disease. 5th edition. Philadelphia: W.B. Saunders; 1994. p. 909–22.
[3] Davidson MB. Diagnosis and classification of diabetes mellitus. In: Davidson MB, editor. Diabetes mellitus—diagnosis and treatment. 3rd edition. New York: Churchill Livingstone; 1991. p. 1–10.
[4] Frykberg RG, Armstrong DG, Giurini J, et al. Diabetic foot disorders: a clinical practice guideline. J Foot Ankle Surg 2000;39(5 Suppl):S1–60.
[5] National Diabetes Data Group. Classification and diagnosis of diabetes mellitus and other categories of glucose intolerance. Diabetes 1979;28(12):1039–57.
[6] Bennett PH. The diagnosis of diabetes: new internal classification and diagnostic criteria. Annu Rev Med 1983;34:295–309.
[7] American Diabetes Association. Report of the Expert Committee on the Diagnosis and Classification of Diabetes Mellitus. Diabetes Care 2001;24:S1–20.
[8] Expert Committee on the Diagnosis and Classification of Diabetes Mellitus. Report of the Expert Committee on the Diagnosis and Classification of Diabetes Mellitus. Diabetes Care 2002;25: S5–20.
[9] Engelgau ME, Narayan KMV, Herman WH. Screening for type 2 diabetes. Diabetes Care 2000; 10:1563–80.
[10] American Diabetes Association. Standards of medical care for patients with diabetes mellitus. Diabetes Care 2002;25:S33–49.
[11] DeFronzo RA, Bonadonna RC, Ferrannini E. Pathogenesis of NIDDM: a balanced overview. Diabetes Care 1992;15:319.
[12] Ludwing DS, Ebbeling CB. Type 2 diabetes mellitus in children; primary care and public health considerations. JAMA 2001;286:1427–30.
[13] American Diabetes Association. Type 2 diabetes in children and adolescents. Diabetes Care 2002; 23:381–9.
[14] Schuster DP, Duvuuri V. Diabetes mellitus. Clin Pod Med Surg 2002;19(1):79–107.
[15] Cudworth AG, Woodrow JC. Genetic susceptibility in diabetes mellitus: analysis of the HLA association. Br Med J 1976;2(6040):846–8.
[16] Overbach D, Naya FJ, Tsai MJ, et al. Analysis of candidate genes for susceptibility to type I diabetes: a case control and family association study of genes on chromosome 2q31–35. Diabetes 1997;46:1069–74.
[17] Forbes LV, Brown LJ, Scott RS. HLA-DQb typing and non-Asp57 alleles in IDDM and non-diabetics subjects in New Zealand. Diabetes Care 1993;2(16):1179–83.

[18] Nepom GT. Immunogenetics and IDDM. Diabetes Rev 1993;1:93.
[19] Yoon JW. Role of viruses in the pathogenesis of IDDM. Ann Intern Med 1991;23:4327.
[20] Szopa TM, Tichener PA, Portwood ND, et al. Diabetes mellitus due to viruses: some recent developments. Diabetelogia 1997;40:53.
[21] Helmke K, Otten A, Willems WR, et al. Islet cell antibodies and the development of diabetes mellitus in relation to mumps infection and mumps vaccination. Diabetologia 1986;29:30–6.
[22] Gerstein HC. Cow's milk exposure and type 1 diabetes mellitus: a critical review of the clinical literature. Diabetes Care 1994;17:13–9.
[23] Kostraba JN, Cruickshanks KJ, Lawler-Heavner J, et al. Early exposure to cow's milk and solid foods in infancy, genetic predisposition and risk of IDDM. Diabetes 1993;42:288–95.
[24] Virtanen SM, et al. Early introduction of dairy products associated with increased risk of IDDM in Finnish children: the Childhood in Diabetes in Finland Study Group. Diabetes 1993;42:1786–90.
[25] Hummel M, Fuchtenbusch M, Schenker M, Ziegler AG. No major association of breast feeding, vaccinations, and childhood viral diseases with early islet autoimmunity in the German BABY-DIAB Study. Diabetes Care 2000;23:969–74.
[26] Takara M, Komiya I, Kinjo Y, et al. Association of CTLA-4 gene A/G polymorphism in Japanese type 1 diabetic patients with younger age of onset and autoimmune thyroid disease. Diabetes Care 2000;23:975–8.
[27] Decochez K, Keymeulen B, Somers G, et al. Use of an islet cell antibody assay to identify type 1 diabetic patients with rapid decrease in c-peptide levels after clinical onset. Diabetes Care 2000;23: 1072–8.
[28] Alberti KGMM. Problems related to definitions and epidemiology of type 2 (non-insulin dependent) diabetes mellitus: studies throughout the world. Diabetologia 1993;36:978–84.
[29] Keller U. Diabetic ketoacidosis: current views on pathogenesis and treatment. Diabetologia 1986;29:71.
[30] Matz R. Hyperosmolar nonacidotic uncontrolled diabetes: not a rare event. Clin Diabetes 1988; 6:25.
[31] Davidson MB. Oral hypoglycemic sulfonylurea agents. In: Davidson MB, editor. Diabetes mellitus—diagnosis and treatment. 3rd edition. New York: Churchill Livingstone; 1991. p. 147–74.
[32] Siconolfi-Baez L, Banerje MA, Lebovitz HE. Characterization and significance of sulfonylurea receptors. Diabetes Care 1990;13:S2–8.
[33] Edelson GW. Pharmacological options for glucose control. Podiatry Today November 1998;11: 54–9.
[34] Shorr RI, Ray WA, Daugherty JR, Griffin MR. Individual sulfonylureas and serious hypoglycemia in older people. J Am Geriatr Soc 1996;44:751–5.
[35] Muhlhauser P, Sawicki T, Berger M. Possible risk of sulfonylureas in the treatment of non-insulin dependent diabetes mellitus and coronary artery disease. Diabetologia 1997;40:1492–6.
[36] Leibowitz G, Cerasi E. Sulfonylurea treatment of NIDDM patients with cardiovascular disease: a mixed blessing. Diabetologia 1996;39:503–14.
[37] Available at: http://www.diabetesnet.com/diabetes-treatments/sulfonylureas.php. website: www.diabetesnet.com. Accessed February 2003.
[38] Available at: http://www.diabetesnet.com/diabetes-treatments/metformin.php. website: www.diabetesnet.com. Accessed February 2003.
[39] Available at: http://www.my.webmd.com/encyclopedia. website: www.diabetesnet.com. Accessed February 2003.
[40] DeFronzo RA. Pharmacological therapy for type 2 diabetes mellitus. Ann Intern Med 1999; 131(4):281–303.
[41] Stumvoll N, Nurjhan N, Perriello G, et al. Metabolic effects of metformin in non-insulin dependent diabetes mellitus. N Engl J Med 1995;333:550–4.
[42] Bailey CJ, Turner RC. Metformin. N Engl J Med 1996;334:54–9.
[43] Misbin RI, Green L, Stadel BV, et al. Lactic acidosis in patients treated with metformin. N Engl J Med 1998;338:265–6.
[44] Available at: http://www.//diabetesnet.com/diabetes-treatments/actos-avandia.php.

[45] Sparanon N, Seaton TL. Troglitazone in type II diabetes mellitus. Pharmacotherapy 1998;18: 539–48.
[46] Raskin P, Jovanovic L, Berger S, et al. Repaglinide/troglitazone combination therapy: improved glycemic control in type 2 diabetes. Diabetes Care 2000;23:979–83.
[47] Einhorn D. Pioglitazone hydrochloride in combination with metformin therapy improves glycemic control in the treatment of patients with type 2 diabetes mellitus: a randomized, placebo-controlled study. Clin Ther 2000;22(12):1395–409.
[48] Warner AL, Travaglini MT. A review of rosiglitazone in type 2 diabetes mellitus. Pharmacotherapy 2001;21:1082–99.
[49] Available at: http://www.diabetesnet.com/diabetes-treatments/precose-glyset.php.
[50] Lebovitz HE. A new oral therapy for diabetes management: alpha-glucosidase inhibition with acarbose. Clin Diabetes 1995;13:99–103.
[51] Kelley DE, Bidot P, Freedman Z, et al. Efficacy and safety of acarbose in insulin-treated patients with type 2 diabetes. Diabetes Care 1998;21:2056–61.
[52] Available at: http://diabetesnet.com/diabetes-treatments/prandin-starlix.php.
[53] Fuhlendorff J, Rorsman P, Kofod H, et al. Stimulation of insulin release by repaglinide and glibenclamide involves both common and distinct processes. Diabetes 1998;47:345–51.
[54] Moses R, Slobodniuk R, Boyages S, et al. Effect of repaglinide addition to metformin monotherapy on glycemic control in patients with type 2 diabetes. Diabetes Care 1999;22:119–24.
[55] GlaxoSmithKline. Avandamet [product insert]. Research Triangle Park (NC): GlaxoSmithKline; 2002.
[56] Bristol-Myers-Squibb. Metaglip [product insert]. Princeton (NJ): Bristol-Myers-Squibb; 2002.
[57] Available at: http://diabetesnet.com/diabetes-treatments/insulin-humalog.php.
[58] Seley JJ. The role of insulin in type 2 diabetes. J Am Acad Phys Assist 2001.
[59] Koivisto VA. Insulin therapy in type II diabetes. Diabetes Care 1993;16:29–39.
[60] Genuth S. Insulin use in NIDDM. Diabetes Care 1990;13:1240–64.
[61] Koivisto VA, Tuominen JA, Ebeling P. Lispro Mix25 insulin as premeal therapy in type 2 diabetic patients. Diabetes Care 1999;22(3):459–62.
[62] Kucera ML, Graham JP. Insulin lispro, a new insulin analog. Pharmacotherapy 1998;18:526–38.
[63] Sindaco PD, Ciofetta M, Lalli C, et al. Use of the short-acting insulin analog lispro in intensive treatment of type 1 diabetes mellitus: importance of appropriate replacement of basal insulin and time-interval injection-meal. Diabet Med 1998;15:592–600.
[64] Bode BW, Strange P. Efficacy, safety, and pump compatibility of insulin aspart used in continuous subcutaneous insulin infusion therapy in patients with type 1 diabetes. Diabetes Care 2001; 24:69–72.
[65] Lindholm A, McEwen J, Riis AP. Improved postprandial glycemic control with insulin aspart. Diabetes Care 1999;22:801–5.
[66] Kang S, Brange J, Burch A, et al. Subcutaneous insulin absorption explained by insulin's physiochemical properties: evidence from absorption studies of soluble human insulin and insulin analogs. Diabetes Care 1991;14:942–8.
[67] Riddle MC, Schneider J. Beginning insulin treatment of obese patients with evening 70/30 insulin plus glimepiride versus insulin alone. Diabetes Care 1998;21:1052–7.
[68] Available at: http://diabetesnet.com/diabetes-treatments/insulin-lantus.php.
[69] McKeage K, Goa KL. Insulin glargine: a review of its therapeutic use as a long-acting agent for the management of type 1 and 2 diabetes mellitus. Drugs 2001;61(11):1599–624.
[70] Rosskamp RH, Park G. Long-acting insulin analogs. Diabetes Care 1999;22:B109–13.
[71] Genuth SM. Treating diabetes with both insulin and sulfonylurea drugs: what is the value? Clin Diabetes 1987;5:74–9.
[72] McCilloch DK, Kurtz AB, Tattersall RB. A new approach to the treatment of nocturnal hypoglycemia using alpha-glucosidase inhibition. Diabetes Care 1983;6:483–7.
[73] Simonson DC, DelPrato S, Castellino P, et al. Effect of glubyride on glycemic control, insulin requirement and glucose metabolism in insulin related diabetic patients. Diabetes 1987;36: 136–46.

[74] Riddle MC, Hart JS, Bouma DJ, et al. Efficacy of bedtime NPH insulin with daytime sulfonylurea for subpopulation of type II diabetic subjects. Diabetes Care 1989;12:623–9.
[75] Trischitta V, Italia S, Borzi V, et al. Low dose bedtime NPH insulin in treatment of secondary failure to glyburide. Diabetes Care 1989;12:582–5.
[76] Landstedt-Hallin L, Adamson U, Arner P, et al. Comparison of bedtime NPH or preprandial regular insulin combined with glibenclamide in secondary sulfonylurea failure. Diabetes Care 1995;18:1183–6.
[77] Shank M, DelPrato S, DeFronzo RA. Bedtime insulin/daytime glipizide. Effective therapy for sulfonylurea failure in NIDDM. Diabetes 1995;44:165–72.
[78] Cusi K, Cunningham GR, Comstock JP. Safety and efficacy of normalizing fasting glucose with bedtime NPH insulin alone in NIDDM. Diabetes Care 1995;18:843–51.
[79] Stratton IM, Adler AI, Neil HA, et al. Association of glycemia with macrovascular and microvascular complications of type 2 diabetes: prospective observational study. BMJ 2000; 321:405–12.
[80] Metchick LN, Petit WA, Inzucchi SE. Inpatient management of diabetes mellitus. Am J Med 2002;113:317–23.
[81] Koivukangas V, Annala AP, Salmela PI, Oikarinen A. Delayed restoration of epidermal barrier function after suction blister injury in patients with diabetes mellitus. Diabet Med 1999;16:563–7.
[82] Inzucchi SE. Glycemic management of diabetes in the perioperative setting. Int Anesthesiol Clin 2002;40:77–93.
[83] Graham GW, Unger BP, Coursin DB. Perioperative management of selected endocrine disorders. Int Anesthesiol Clin 2000;38:31–67.
[84] Hirsch IB, McGill JB. Role of insulin in management of surgical patients with diabetes mellitus. Diabetes Care 1990;13:980–91.
[85] Pezzarossa A, Taddei F, Cimicchi MC, et al. Perioperative management of diabetic subjects. Subcutaneous versus intravenous insulin administration during glucose-potassium infusion. Diabetes Care 1988;11(1):52–8.
[86] Husband DJ, Thai AC, Alberti KGMM. Management of diabetes during surgery with glucose-insulin-potassium infusion. Diabet Med 1986;3:69–74.
[87] Popp DA, Tse TF, Shah S, et al. Oral propranolol and metoprolol both impair glucose recovery from insulin induced hypoglycemia in insulin dependent diabetes mellitus. Diabetes Care 1984;7: 243–7.
[88] Amiel SA, Gale E. Physiological responses to hypoglycemia: counterregulation and cognitive function. Diabetes Care 1993;16:S48–55.
[89] Cryer PE. Hypoglycemia unawareness in IDDM. Diabetes Care 1993;16.
[90] Mazze RS, Lucido D, Shamoon H. Psychological and social correlates of glycemic control. Diabetes Care 1984;7:360–6.
[91] Gavard JA, Lustman PJ, Clouse RE. Prevalence of depression in adults with diabetes: an epidemiological evaluation. Diabetes Care 1993;16:1167–78.

Clin Podiatr Med Surg
20 (2003) 655–669

CLINICS IN
PODIATRIC
MEDICINE AND
SURGERY

Diabetic foot infections and antibiotic therapy

Thomas Zgonis, DPM[a,*], Gary Peter Jolly, DPM[b],
Benjamin J. Buren, DPM[c], Peter Blume, DPM[d]

[a]*The Center for Reconstructive Foot Surgery, 440 New Britain Avenue, Plainville, CT 06062, USA*
[b]*New Britain General Hospital, New Britain, CT 06052, USA*
[c]*West Haven-Yale Podiatric Surgery, USA*
[d]*Department of Orthopaedics and Rehabilitation, Yale University School of Medicine, New Haven, CT 06510, USA*

Diabetic foot infections are the most common cause of lower extremity amputations. Diabetic neuropathy, angiopathy, renal disease, and multisystem failure are some of the factors that can lead to a limb or a life-threatening infection and subsequent amputation. Soft tissue or bone infections in diabetics are usually managed surgically, supplemented by antibiotic therapy and vascular reconstruction when appropriate. All necrotic and infected soft tissue or bone should be removed from the wound, thereby converting the defect to a surgically clean acute wound. Antibiotic therapy should begin with a drug, such as cefazolin, which provides excellent coverage against staphylococci and streptococci. It is only after deep cultures are taken during surgery that definitive antibiotic therapy can begin. The duration of treatment can be variable, lasting from 1 week for mild infections to more than 6 weeks in cases of osteomyelitis and severe deep tissue infection. Aggressive surgical intervention and appropriate antibiotic therapy will reduce the likelihood of major amputations and the duration of hospitalization [1].

A detailed history and physical examination is the most important subset of information available to the physician. A history of puncture wounds, burns, or other trauma should raise the index of suspicion for infection. Nausea, vomiting, uncontrolled blood glucose levels, sweating, fever, red streaking, and open sores are important findings as well. Chronic ulcers with exposed bone, sinus tracks, drainage of purulent material, malodor, and pain in an otherwise neuropathic foot are most definite signs of a diabetic foot infection.

In a study done by Grayson et al [2], the ability to probe to bone in the base of an ulcer with a sterile blunt steel probe had a positive predictive value of 89% and a negative predictive value of 56%. This test should be employed in the assessment

* Corresponding author.
E-mail address: thomaszgonis@yahoo.com (T. Zgonis).

doi:10.1016/S0891-8422(03)00067-3

of all foot ulcers that appear infected, and may obviate further radiographic tests to confirm the diagnosis of osteomyelitis.

Laboratory tests may not be as useful in the initial diagnosis of infections in diabetic patients because a leukocytosis may be absent or only modest at best in these patients. Initial tests should include a complete blood count and differential, electrolytes, blood urea nitrogen, creatinine, glucose levels, and erythrocyte sedimentation rate. Sedimentation rates above 70 mm/h may suggest the presence of osteomyelitis [3]. Blood cultures, urinalysis, radiographs of the foot, tissue cultures and gram stain, and further radiological testing should also be considered depending on the severity of the diabetic foot infection and the course of intervention being considered.

Superficial cultures taken by swab of an ulcer bed will contain colonized bacteria, not necessarily the infecting organism or organisms. Deep tissue samples or bone scrapings are more reliable specimens for harvesting cultures [4]. A study by Pellizzer et al [5] compared the reliability between ulcer swabbing and deep tissue biopsy in 29 diabetic patients with limb-threatening foot infections. The mean number of isolates per patient was found to be 2.34 by swabbing and 2.07 by tissue biopsy sampling. No statistical significance could be shown between the two methods of culturing, but deep tissue cultures were found to be more sensitive than swabbing for monitoring isolates with antibiotic resistance.

Imaging

Soft tissue infections that are uncomplicated by abscess formation, tendon sheath involvement, or bone and joint involvement will generally respond to an appropriate course of antibiotics. When there is a suspicion of an underlying bone infection, confirmation of those suspicions can be problematic at times, particularly when there is either a preexisting or an acute Charcot deformity in progress. Radiographs of such a patient may make it impossible to determine whether the underlying bone may be compromised by an infection.

Because of the destructive changes associated with Charcot neuroarthropathy, standard radiographs offer little in diagnosing an underlying osteomyelitis. A controversy exists in the literature over the best imaging techniques to distinguish osteomyelitis from Charcot neuroarthropathy [6–8]. It is the authors' position that the ability to probe to bone and the presence of clinical and systemic signs of infection is still the most reliable indicator of the presence of osteomyelitis. Grayson et al [2] showed that probing to bone in infected pedal ulcers in patients with diabetes was strongly correlated with the presence of underlying osteomyelitis (66%), and that radionuclide tests and other medical imaging tests might not be necessary to confirm the diagnosis of osteomyelitis when an examiner can touch exposed bone.

Imaging techniques commonly used in the confirmation of osteomyelitis include plain radiographs, scintigraphy, magnetic resonance imaging, computerized tomography, and diagnostic ultrasound. Each test has its own set of limitations, and careful patient evaluation is necessary before ordering an expensive and possibly unnecessary test. Plain radiographs are usually taken at the initial visit and are the baseline by which to monitor any destructive process of bone. An initial radiolucency that develops from an underlying osteomyelitis requires between 5 and 7 days to be seen, and 10 to 14 days for the first signs of sequestrum and involucrum to be noticeable. Osseous changes on plain radiographs may be detected when there has been a 35% to 50% reduction in bone mineral density in comparison with the surrounding bone stock. Radiographs are easily available, inexpensive, and can be used to determine the presence of soft tissue swelling, gas in the tissues, cortical irregularity, periosteal reaction, and focal demineralization [9]. Radiographs with osteomyelits will be abnormal in less than 5% of the patients on early presentation, but by the third or fourth week 90% of the patients will demonstrate clinical changes consistent with osteomyelitis [10].

Scintigraphy is used to confirm the diagnosis of osteomyelitis and to determine its extent. Technesium-99 bone scans can be positive for osteomyelitis, neuropathic osteoarthropathy, fractures, tumors, arthritides, and postsurgical changes, so it is not specific but is sensitive for the diagnosis of osteomyelitis. Devillers et al [11] compared the efficacy of Tc-99m-labeled antigranulocyte monoclonal antibody fragment Fab' (Leukoscan) scintigraphy versus Tc-99m-labeled leukocyte scintigraphy (HMPAO-LS) for the diagnosis of unselected patients with bone and joint infection. In their study, the overall sensitivity, specificity, and accuracy were 86%, 72%, and 78%, respectively, for Leukoscan scintigraphy and 93%, 100%, and 96%, respectively, for HMPAO-LS scans. HMPAO-LS scintigraphy was proven to be more specific than Leukoscan scintigraphy in detecting bone infection in the diabetic foot [11]. Gallium-67, Indium-111, Tec-99 HMPAO, and sulfur colloid scans have all been used to confirm the diagnosis of osteomyelitis [12,13].

Magnetic resonance imaging may also be useful to confirm the diagnosis of osteomyelitis [14–17]. Postsurgical changes, Charcot neuroarthropathy, trauma, fractures, and avascular necrosis may generate false positives. Ledermann et al [18] used contrast-enhanced MR imaging to evaluate the frequency, distribution, and extent of tendon involvement in patients with pedal infection and concluded that through MR imaging, detection of tendon infection could influence the plan of surgical therapy. In a different study by the aforementioned author, a contrast material-enhanced MR imaging was used to document the expected frequency, location, and size of pedal abcesses. The study showed that abscesses are significantly more frequent in patients with osteomyelitis and in feet that have had previous surgery and that magnetic resonance imaging was useful in detecting osteomyelitis [19].

The use of CT scans and ultrasound imaging to confirm the diagnosis of osteomyelitis is promising, but they still have limitations. Enderle et al [20] studied the efficacy of ultrasound in the diagnosis of osteomyelitis in the diabetic foot and compared it to MRI, bone scintigraphy, and plain film radiography. The sensitivity, specificity, positive predictive value, and negative predictive value was found to be 79%, 80%, 92%, and 57% respectively for ultrasound; 69%, 80%, 90%, and 50% respectively for plain film radiography; 83%, 75%, 91%, and 60% respectively for bone scintigraphy; and 100%, 75%, 93%, and 100% respectively for MRI. The study showed that ultrasound was superior of plain films for detecting chronic osteomyelitis in the diabetic foot and has similar sensitivity and specificity with bone scans. However, MRI was superior to all other methods [20].

A definitive diagnosis of osteomyelitis can only be made by bone biopsy with culture and histological analysis. Bone specimens can be obtained in surgery or percutaneously under fluoroscopic imaging. Bone cultures should be obtained if there is a high index of suspicion for underlying osteomyelitis and the results from imaging are inconclusive.

Common pathogens

In mild diabetic foot infections with no previous antibiotic therapy and in the absence of any acute systemic symptoms, gram-positive aerobic cocci are the most common pathogens encountered, specifically *Staphylococcus aureus* followed by aerobic streptococci. Severe, life-threatening infections generally present with polymicrobial infections, including Pseudomonas aureginosa, Enterobacteriaceae, anaerobes such as Bacteroides, Peptococcus, Peptostreptococcus, Clostridium, Fusobacterium, Enterococcus, methicillin-resistant staphylococci, and vancomycin-resistant enterococci. Definitive therapy must include an antibiotic regimen that will provide coverage for all of the infecting organisms.

Antibiotic agents

Most diabetic foot infections are treated empirically until cultures and sensitivities are finalized. It should be presumed that either staphylococcus or streptococcus is present, so that the initial agent chosen should provide coverage for these organisms. Oral therapy for a superficial soft tissue infection, which has not produced fever, leukoytosis, or significant elevations in the patient's glucose level, may be appropriate. For deeper or limb-threatening infections, an empiric regimen should be initiated to cover the most common pathogens, including gram-negative bacilli and anaerobes. In these patients, it is usually staphylococcus or streptococcus that produces the systemic response of fever and leukocytosis, so the drug of choice should provide coverage against staph and strep and in sufficiently high serum and tissue levels. Cefazolin or sublactam/sodium penicillins are excellent choices for initial coverage while waiting for definitive cultures. Empiric therapy should be only changed if there is worsening of the clinical picture. If there is clinical improvement, the empiric regimen should be maintained, and if the definitive culture contains resistant organisms, additional antibiotics may be added to the treatment. Frequently changing antibiotic therapy can create resistant pathogens that require more complex antibiotic combinations. If clinical improvement is not observed while the patient is on empiric antibiotic therapy, then surgical intervention in the form of incision and drainage and adequate debridement may be indicated.

The dosage and duration of intravenous versus oral antibiotic therapy in diabetic foot infections is not completely clear. For mild or superficial infections oral antibiotics might be adequate for 1 to 2 weeks, but for systemically ill patients with severe infections, intravenous therapy is necessary. Patients with vascular disease, end-stage renal disease, hypertension, and liver disease need to be carefully evaluated before administering long-term antibiotics. Topical antibiotics have no real place in the treatment of diabetic foot infections and may produce the development of resistant strains of colonized surface bacteria [21,22]. Absorbable antibiotic impregnated calcium sulfate pellets have been used in patients with osteomyelitis and may be used adjunctively in the management of diabetic bone infections [23].

The choice of antibiotics should be based on culture and susceptibility tests. An intraoperative bone culture is preferable, but if this is not immediately available, an empiric therapy should be initiated with an eye toward coverage of staph or strep. Mild or superficial diabetic infections without bone or deep tissue involvement can usually be managed by a single antimicrobial agent. Oral therapy may be started with cephalexin, 500 mg every 6 hours; dicloxacillin, 500 mg to 1 g every 6 hours; clindamycin, 300 mg every 6 hours; amoxicillin/clavulanate, 500 mg every 8 hours or 875 mg every 12 hours; cefadroxil, 1 g every 12 hours; levofloxacin, 500 mg or 750 mg once a day; and ciprofloxacin, 750 mg every 12 hours.

Intravenous (IV) therapy include nafcillin or oxacillin, 2 g every 4 hours; cefazolin, 1 to 2 g every 8 hours; cefepime, 2 g every 12 hours; clindamycin, 600 mg every 6 to 8 hours; and ampicillin/sulbactam, 3 g every 6 hours. In cases of methicillin-resistant staphylococci (MRSA), the following pharmacotherapy should be considered: vancomycin IV, 1g every 12 hours; linezolid IV or PO, 600 mg every 12 hours; and quinopristin/dalfopristin, 7.5 mg/kg every 12 hours. Patients with a true allergy to penicillin or penicillin derivatives should be administered oral therapy of clindamycin or fluoroquinolones and intravenous therapy of vancomycin or clindamycin.

Cephalexin is a first-generation cephalosporin and provides better coverage for gram-positive cocci, with the exception of methicillin-resistant strains of staph. The mechanism of action of cephalosporins appears to be similar to that of the penicillins and is contraindicated to patients with a known beta-lactam allergy. In patients with renal disease, the dose should be decreased based on the patient's renal function. Probenecid increases serum levels and side effects include diarrhea and interstitial nephritis. Dicloxacillin is a penicillinase-resistant penicillin with good gram-positive coverage, but is not effective against methicillin-resistant strains. It is also contraindicated in patients with a beta-lactam allergy. Clindamycin is an antianaerobic agent that also provides coverage against gram-positive cocci (except MRSA), *Enterococcus* and *Clostridium* species. It has no activity against aerobic gram-negative bacilli and is used in patients with a known penicillin or cephalosporin allergy. Side effects include diarrhea and antibiotic-associated colitis and hepatic impairment. Amoxicillin/clavulanate (Augmentin) is a beta lactamase inhibitor that may be useful in treating gram-positive cocci, but it possesses no coverage of pseudomonas, serratia, citrobacter, or enterobacter. It also covers gram-negative cocci and anaerobes, including bacteroides. Amoxicillin/clavulanate is contraindicated in patients with a known beta-lactam allergy and side effects include diarrhea, intersitial nephritis, elevation of liver enzymes, and bone marrow suppression. Cefadroxil is a first-generation cephalosporin that is similar to cephalexin, but its dosing and frequency are less than that of cephalexin.

The fluoroquinolones are a group of antibiotics that include ciprofloxacin and levofloxacin. As a class they are contraindicated in pregnant women or patients who are younger than 16 years. They have good gram-negative coverage and excellent bone penetration but are less active against staphylococci and anaerobes. Their use in monotherapy in diabetic foot infections are therefore inappropriate, but in combination with a cephalosporin, clindamycin, or a penicillin/clavulonate are effective. Fluoroquinolone tablets have a 100% bioavailability comparing favorably to the intravenous administration of these drugs. Side effects of the fluoroquinolones include gastrointestinal discomfort, reported tendon ruptures, prolonged QT intervals, nausea, headaches, and insomnia [24]. Certain precautions in patients taking theophylline, antacids, caffeine products, diazepam, probenecid, and iron supplements should be taken. Nix and associates [25] were the first to demonstrate successful treatment of serious soft tissue or bone infections with oral ciprofloxacin alone, and 79% of their patients were treated without the need of amputation.

A prospective randomized multicenter study by Lipsky et al [26] compared the efficacy of parenteral ofloxacin followed by oral ofloxacin and intravenous ampicillin/sublactam followed by amoxicillin/clavulanate) and showed that a 3-week therapy with either regimen was effective in treating the diabetic foot infections in 108 patients with 24% of osteomyelitis cases. A study by Sesin et al [27] showed the efficacy of an oral combination of clindamycin and ciprofloxacin therapy for diabetic foot infections. The use of their oral antimicrobial agents significantly reduced the duration of the patients' hospital stay and increased the cost savings. In another recent prospective study by Goldstein et al [28], an increased prevalence of MRSA and Enterococci in diabetic foot infections along with a resistance to levofloxacin and sparfloxacin was noted.

Siami et al [29] performed a randomized study involving 409 patients with severe skin and soft tissue infections who were being treated with either clinafloxacin or piperacillin-tazobactam. *Staphylococcus aureus*, *Enterococcus faecalis*, and *Pseudomonas aeruginosa* were the most commonly encountered pathogens. They concluded from their study that clinafloxacin was just as effective as piperacillin-tazobactam in the treatment of severe skin and soft tissue infection in this patient population. Senneville et al [30] showed a cure rate of 88.2% with combined antibiotic therapy consisting of ofloxacin and rifampicin in the treatment of mild to moderate diabetic foot osteomyelitis. Rissing [31] showed that quinolones were effective in chronic osteomyelitis with appropriate surgery and adequate duration of therapy.

Vancomycin is active against methicillin-resistant staphylococcus, enterococci, Clostridium, and most of the gram-positive cocci. Some of the side effects seen with this drug include nephrotoxicity, ototoxicity, hypersensitivity, and thrombophlebitis at the IV site. The dosage and the frequency of dosage of vancomycin are determined by the patient's body weight and renal function. Serum trough levels of vancomycin are determined initially and subsequent doses are titrated accordingly. Vancomycin is a good alternative for staph and strep coverage in patients with a known penicillin or cephalosporin allergy.

Linezolid (Zyvox) is the first antibiotic in a new class called the oxazolidinones. They have a unique mechanism of action whereby they interfere with ribosomal initiation complex formation [32,33]. Cross-resistance with existing antimicrobials is unlikely. The spectrum of activity includes clinically important gram-positive pathogens. It can be administered parenterally and orally. The indications for linezolid include VRE faecium infections/bacteremia, hospital-acquired pneumonia, complicated and uncomplicated skin and skin structure infections, and community acquired pneumonia. The spectrum of in vitro activity of linezolid includes many gram-positive microorganisms, including, but not limited to, *Staphylococcus aureus*, *Staphylococcus pneumoniae*, *Staphylococcus pyogenes*, *Staphylococcus agalactae*, and *enterococcus faecalis* (including vancomycin-resistant strains), in addition to staphphylococcus epidermidis, methicillin-resistant strains, and viridans group streptococcus. There have been approximately eight pivotal studies in summation with the FDA, including seven randomized multicenter comparative trials and one open-label trial [34,35]. Linezolid is administered as a 600 mg IV injection every 12 hours, and the same for the oral preparation. The pharmacokinetics of Linezolid in the geriatric population will not require dose adjustment. Linezolid is not indicated for pediatric patients. The excretion of linezolid is through the urine as a direct and indirect metabolite. There is no dose adjustment recommended for renal impairment, including those on hemodialysis. There is no dose adjustment for mild to moderate hepatic impairment. Linezolid does inhibit monoamine oxidase and may interact with adrenergic agents and large quantities of tyramine-containing foods. There is no interaction with gentamicin, aztreonam were agents metabolized by cytochrome p450 isoforms. There is no apparent interaction with warfarin (Coumadin) or phenytoin (Dilantin). This drug is a superb for methicillin-resistant staph aureus infections and can be treated with PO preparations at 600 mg twice daily. The bioavailability of the oral linezolid is equal to or better than the parenteral counterpart. Linezolid is unique when compared with vancomycin because it is 100% orally bioavailable. Linezolid is as effective as vancomycin in the treatment of complicated skin and skin structure infections and ammonia due to MRSA. Safety considerations should include careful observation for myelosuppression (anemia, leukopenia, pancytopenia, and thrombocytopenia). Discontinuation of therapy will allow for reversal of this hematologic change. The most frequent adverse events typically include diarrhea, headache, nausea, vomiting, and constipation. This drug enables the practitioner to avoid long-term peripheral intravenous central catheter placement and the associated complications of thrombophlebitis and line sepsis. This drug should be reserved for those with documented and cultured methicillin-resistant staph aureus infections.

Ertapenem (Invanz) is a new parenteral Carbapenem within our spectrum and imipenem or Meropenem. Carbapenems are beta-lactam antibiotics. They inhibit cell wall synthesis in a similar manner to penicillins and cephalosporins. Unlike penicillin and cephalosporins, they are resistant to hydrolysis by beta-lactamase, including extended spectrum beta-lactamase. Ertapenem has been compared with Zosyn in 540 adults with comparable clinical efficacy and tolerability. It is indicated for moderate to severe complicated skin and skin structure infections. It has a similar effectiveness to that of ticarcillin/clavulanic acid, ampicillin/sulbactam, and cefoxitin or cefotetan with or without an aminoglycoside. Ertapenem is contraindicated in patients with known hypersensitivity to beta-lactams. The intramuscular dose with lidocaine hydrochloride as a diluent may also present a hypersensitivity. The most common drug-related adverse experiences were diarrhea, infused vein complications, nausea, and headache. The dosage for Ertapenem is 1 g per day IV or IM. Patients with advanced renal insufficiency or end-stage renal disease should receive 500 mg per day. Ertapenem may be administered by intravenous infusion for up to 14 days or intramuscularly for up to 7 days. It should be infused over a 30-minute period. Ertapenem is a broad-spectrum, well-tolerated drug with once-daily dosing. It is suitable as a first-line empiric monotherapy. It has better anaerobic coverage than Rocephin. It has extensive and excellent anaerobic coverage. It has fewer daily doses than Zosyn and other drugs used to treat anaerobes. It is an excellent choice for home IV antibiotic therapy with excellent clinical efficacy for moderate to severe complicated skin and skin structure infections.

Quinopristin/dalfopristin (Synercid) is a new drug, recently made available by the FDA, which is active against MRSA and vancomycin-resistant enterococci (VRE). MRSA colonization of chronic foot ulcers is a cause of MRSA bacteremia and an increasingly frequent problem, which needs to be treated aggressively [36–38]. Lautenbach et al [39] showed that restricting the frequency of use of vancomycin and third-generation cephalosporins had little impact on VRE prevalence and that clindamycin was associated with the development of VRE more frequently than vancomycin.

Deep, soft tissue infections with or without involvement of bone in diabetics requires an aggressive surgical debridement and adequate antibiotic therapy. Adequate blood flow is required to produce sufficient tissue levels of the antibiotics in the bone and soft tissue if the antimicrobial is to be effective. Parenteral therapy is always initiated in these conditions for better soft tissue and bone penetration. Antimicrobial agents include ampicillin/sulbactam, 3 g every 6 hours; ticarcillin/clavulanate, 3.1 g every 6 hours; pipercillin/tazobactam, 3.375 or 4.5 g every 8 hours; clindamycin, 600 mg IV every 6 hours and ciprofloxacin, 400 mg IV or 750 mg PO every 12 hours; cefoxitin, 1.5 to 2 g IV every 6 hours; cefepime, 2 g IV every 12 hours; ceftazidime, 2 g IV every 8 hours; and ceftriaxone, 2 g IV daily plus metronidazole 500 mg PO or IV every 6 hours. For deeper soft tissue infections without bone involvement, parenteral therapy is recommended initially for 7 to 10 days, followed by 3 to 4 weeks of oral therapy. The duration of therapy for osteomyelitis, even though there is no clinical data to support it, is 4 to 6 weeks of intravenous therapy. If all of the necrotic and infected bone has been surgically removed, then treatment may be reduced to 2 weeks of parenteral therapy followed by a total of 6 weeks of oral antibiotics. If surgical debridement was not performed, then a 4- to 6-week parenteral course followed by 2 months of oral therapy is indicated [40]. The duration of treatment for osteomyelitis a rather contentious issue and is likely to remain one until definitive outcome data becomes available. A study by Venkatesan et al [41] showed that a conservative regimen of oral antibiotics given for an average of 27 months was adequate to manage osteomyelitis in the diabetic foot. In their study, 17 out of 22 patients resolved their osteomyelitis with oral clindamycin alone [41].

Ampicillin/sulbactam (Unasyn), ticarcillin/clavulanate (Timentin), and pipercillin/tazobactam (Zosyn) are beta-lactamase inhibitor agents that are given intravenously. They are active against staphylococci except MRSA; anaerobes, including Bacteroides; and most gram-negative organisms. A study by Klepser et al [42] compared the bacteriocidal activities of the aforementioned drugs against clinical isolates of *Bacteroides fragilis*, *Enterococcus faecalis*, *E coli*, and *Pseudomonas aeruginosa*. They found that all the regimens showed good activity against *B fragilis* and *E coli* but provided a bactericidal activity of less than 50% against *E faecalis* and *P aureginosa* [42].

Beta-lactamase inhibitors are not indicated in patients with penicillin allergy and their main side effects include anaphylaxis, diarrhea, thrombophlebitis at infusion site, bone marrow suppression, and reduced platelet function. Dose adjustment is necessary in patients with renal disease. Beta-lactamase inhibitors are a good choice for polymicrobial infections or infections with resistant nosocomial organisms. Zeillemaker et al [43] showed that piperacillin/tazobactam was more effective for monotherapy in diabetic foot infections than other broad-spectrum antibiotics. File and Tan [44] reported on the efficacy of ticarcillin/clavulanate as monotherapy for bacterial skin and soft tissue infections. Akova et al [45], in a prospective study of 74 patients, demonstrated that ampicillin-sulbactam had clinical cure rates of 86% in patients with osteomyelitis and 100% in patients with soft tissue infections. The most common side effect associated with the use of this drug was diarrhea (14%).

Cefoxitin is a second-generation cephalosporin and is active against anaerobes, including Bacteroides. It has greater coverage of gram-negative organisms than cefazolin, but is less active against gram-positive organisms. Cefepime is a fourth-generation cephalosporin that has excellent coverage of gram-positive and gram-negative organisms. Ceftazidime and ceftriaxone are third-generation cephalosporins, which provide good gram-negative coverage. Ceftazidime is capable of producing high tissue concentrations, even in ischemic limbs, and it is for this reason that it is often used [46]. Ceftriaxone is eliminated by the biliary system and there is a higher incidence of diarrhea with its use than with ceftazidime. Ceftazidime is also the most active cephalosporin against pseudomonas. Metronidazole (Flagyl) has excellent activity against gram-negative anaerobes, including Bacteroides, but is ineffective against aerobic bacteria. Side effects produced by metronidazole include dry mouth with a metallic taste, gastric discomfort, and headaches. It is contraindicated during pregnancy or with alcohol consumption.

Limb or life-threatening infections are surgical emergencies that need to be addressed quickly and aggressively. Antimicrobial regimens include imipenem, 500 mg every 6 hours; meropenem, 1 g every 8 hours; clindamycin, 900 mg IV every 8 hours plus cirpofloxacin 400 mg IV every 12 hours or ceftazidime 2 g IV every 8 hours; pipercillin/tazobactam 3.375 g or ticarcillin/clavulanate, 3.1 g every 4 hours; vancomycin, 1 g every 12 hours plus aztreonam 2 g IV every 8 hours plus metronidazole 500 mg IV every 6 hours; vancomycin 1 g IV every 12 hours plus cefepime 2 g IV every 12 hours; and ceftazidime 2 g IV every 8 hours plus metronidazole 500 mg IV every 6 hours. In this group, parenteral and oral therapy is prolonged and is determined by the outcome and severity of the infection.

Imipenem is a monobactam and is the drug of choice for this infection. It is also indicated for treatment of resistant infections or as an alternative in treating polymicrobial infections. Imipenem and imipenem/cilastin (Primaxin) are contraindicated in patients with a history of seizure disorders. Side effects of imipenem include diarrhea, bone marrow suppression, anaphylaxis, fever, nausea, and phlebitis at the infusion site. Dose adjustments are necessary in patients with renal disease because the drug is cleared through the kidneys. Aztreonam (Azactam) is a monobactam, has a narrow spectrum against gram-negative bacilli, and is a good choice in combination with vancomycin or clindamycin. Some of the newer monobactams include meropenem (Merrem) and ertapenem (Invanz). A double-blind randomized study done by Grayson et al [47] showed the same efficacy of ampicillin/sulbactam compared with imipenem/cilastin for the empirical and definitive treatment of limb-threatening diabetic foot infections.

Suggested empiric therapy for diabetic foot infections

Diabetic foot infections can vary in severity and therefore in antibiotic usage and duration. Severe infections require hospitalization, surgical debridement, and prolonged use of intravenous antibiotics. Mild infections can be treated with outpatient surgery and adequate oral antibiotic therapy. In both situations, an adequate blood supply and adequate management of the patient's comorbidities is necessary to obtain a successful outcome.

Antibiotic combinations that are synergistic can be of great clinical value in the management of patients with diabetic foot infections. Pathare and Sathe [48] reported on a study involving 272 patients, and their results showed that amongst 14 drug combinations tested, four were found to be most effective in treating diabetic foot infections. These included amikacin and piperacillin (77.5%); ampicillin and sulbactam/pipercillin 76.92%; ampicillin/sulbactam and cefoperazone (74.47%), and ofloxacillin and cefotaxime (71.43%). Diamantopoulos et al [49] evaluated the bacteriological and clinical efficacy of the combination of ciprofloxacin and clindamycin in severe diabetic foot infections. Initial empirical antibiotic therapy with ciprofloxacin given in 300 mg doses every 12 hours intravenously and clindamycin given in 600 mg doses every 8 hours intravenously was studied in 84 hospitalized diabetics with severe lower limb infections. The long-term follow-up (mean 16 months) revealed that combination therapy with ciprofloxacin and clindamycin was an excellent empirical combination because of the broad range of coverage, and was effective as a definitive treatment of severe diabetic foot infections [49].

In patients with severe diabetic foot infections, an empiric antibiotic regimen should be initiated and definite therapy should be started when the culture and sensitivities are available. Infected or necrotic bone should be removed from the diabetic ulcer and cultured for more accurate results.

Surgery and infected wounds

Wound debridement should be aggressive with the intention of removing all necrotic bone and soft tissue. It is also essential to ensure that adequate perfusion of the limb is provided to allow for tissue repair and to facilitate the delivery of adequate tissue levels of antibiotics. Seabrook and associates found that inadequate tissue concentrations of many antibiotics were found in amputated limbs and debrided tissue, despite adequate serum levels. They concluded that debridement of devitalized tissue was essential for achieving adequate tissue levels of antibiotics [50].

Debridement may take several forms in the diabetic foot. There is often a tendency on the part of the surgeon, often at the behest of the patient, to try to "save" as much of the foot as possible. Nehler et al [51] studied the intermediate success and outcome of primary forefoot amputations in patients with diabetes mellitus who had sepsis limited to the forefoot and presumed adequate forefoot perfusion, as determined by means of noninvasive methods. Their conclusions were that patients with diabetes mellitus who had sepsis limited to the forefoot requiring acute hospitalization and undergoing primary digit amputations had a high incidence of intermediate-term, persistent, and recurrent infection, leading to a modest rate of limb loss, despite having apparently salvageable lesions and noninvasive evidence of presumed adequate forefoot perfusion [51]. Therefore, a more proximal level of debridement or amputation is likely to provide a reduced risk of recurrent infections in the foot.

Bamberger et al [52] demonstrated in their retrospective study that many patients without extensive necrosis respond to high-dose intravenous antibiotics and may not require amputation to halt infection. Lipsky et al [53] showed that uncomplicated lower extremity infections in patients with DM responded well to outpatient management with oral antibiotic therapy alone.

Recommendations

Diabetes is a strong predictor of mortality related to infection [54]. Infected diabetic wounds and osteomyelitis can lead to a lower extremity amputation and be a major source of disability and morbidity. Severe diabetic foot infections should be treated aggressively by adequate surgical debridement, vascular reconstruction when indicated, appropriate antibiotic therapy, management of the patient's comorbidities, adjuctive local wound care, and off-loading. Paramount to the successful treatment of diabetic infections is a well-educated and compliant patient.

We would be remiss not to at least briefly mention the cost of treating diabetic foot infections. Unfortunately, a good deal of the expenses associated with this subset of patients may be incurred unnecessarily. A study by Eckman et al [55] showed that a significant fraction of the expense in treating diabetic foot infections was incurred from imaging studies that had little or no impact on treatment regimens or patient outcomes. They demonstrated that for patients with deep soft tissue infection and clinical suspicion of osteomyelitis but without evidence of systemic toxicity, a 10-week course of culture-guided oral antibiotic therapy had similar efficacy and lower costs than the conventional approach to management, involving a diagnostic workup in an attempt to establish whether osteomyelitis was present [55]. Local standards of care are likely to drive diagnostic and therapeutic decisions, but as pressures from managed care organizations increase, the current decision-making processes are likely to be critically examined through the filters of future outcome studies.

Summary

Diabetic foot infections are associated with high morbidity and mortality rates as well as significant financial impact on the health care system. Improved patient outcomes and intelligent use of resources should determine the selection of diagnostic procedures and the therapeutic modalities used. Diabetic patients who develop lower extremity infections require a multidisciplinary approach in the management of their infections and other disorders. Aggressive surgical debridement and appropriate and adequate antibiotic therapy are necessary to successfully treat severe foot infections and permit faster recovery.

References

[1] Tan JS, Fiedman NM, Hazelton-Miller C, et al. Can aggressive treatment of diabetic foot infections reduce the need for above-ankle amputation? Clin Infect Dis 1996;23:286–91.
[2] Grayson ML, Gibbons GW, Balogh K, et al. Probing to bone in infected pedal ulcers: a clinical sign of underlying osteomyelitis in diabetic patients. JAMA 1995;273:721–3.
[3] Kaleta JL, Fleischli JW, Reilly CH. The diagnosis of osteomyelitis in diabetes using the erythrocyte sedimentation rate: a pilot study. J Am Podiatr Med Assoc 2001;91:445–50.
[4] Lipsky BA, Pecoraro RE, Wheat JL. The diabetic foot: soft tissue and bone infection. Infect Dis Clin North Am 1990;4:409–32.
[5] Pellizzer G, Strazzabosco M, Presi S, et al. Deep tissue biopsy vs. superficial swab culture monitoring in the microbiological assessment of limb-threatening diabetic foot infection. Diabet Med 2001;18:822–7.
[6] Newman LG. Imaging techniques in the diabetic foot. Clin Podiatr Med Surg 1995;12:75–86.

[7] Harvey J, Cohen MM. Technesium-99 labeled leukocytes in diagnosing diabetic osteomyelitis in the foot. J Foot Ankle Surg 1997;36:209–14.
[8] Craig JG, Amin MB, Wu W, et al. Osteomyelitis of the diabetic foot: MR imaging-pathologic correlation. Radiology 1997;203:849–55.
[9] Bonakdarpour A, Gaines VD. The radiology of osteomyelitis. Orthop Clin North Am 1983;14: 21–37.
[10] Wheat J. Diagnostic strategies in osteomyelitis. Am J Med 1985;78:218–24.
[11] Devillers A, Garin E, Polard JL, et al. Comparison of Tc-99m-labelled antileukocyte fragment Fab' and Tc-99m-HMPAO leukocyte scintigraphy in the diagnosis of bone and joint infections: a prospective study. Nucl Med Commun 2000;2:747–53.
[12] Blume PA, Dey HM, Daley LJ, et al. Diagnosis of pedal osteomyelitis with Tec-99m HMPAO labeled leukocytes. J Foot Ankle Surg 1997;36:120–6.
[13] Larcos G, Brown ML, Sutton RT. Diagnosis of osteomyelitis of the foot in diabetic patients: value of 111 In-leukocyte scintigraphy. AJR Am J Roentgenol 1991;157:527–31.
[14] Cook TA, Rahim N, Sompson HCR, Gelland RB. Magnetic resonance imaging in the management of diabetic foot infection. Br J Surg 1996;83:245–8.
[15] Lipman BT, Collier BD, Carrera GF, et al. Detection of osteomyelitis in the neuropathic foot: nuclear medicine, MRI and conventional radiology. Clin Nucl Med 1998;23:77–82.
[16] Mason MD, Zlatkin MB, Esterhai JL, et al. Chronic complicated osteomyelitis of the lower extremity evaluation with MR imaging. Radiology 1989;173:355–9.
[17] Ledermann HP, Morrision WB, Schweitzer ME, Raikin SM. Tendon involvement in pedal infection: MR analysis of frequency, distribution, and spread of infection. AJR Am J Roentgenol 2002;179:939–47.
[18] Ledermann HP, Morrison WB, Schweitzer ME. Pedal abscesses in patients suspected of having pedal osteomyelitis: analysis with MR imaging. Radiology 2002;224:649–55.
[19] Ledermann HP, Schweitzer ME, Morrison WB. Nonenhancing tissue on MR imaging of pedal infection: characterization of necrotic tissue and associated limitation for diagnosis of osteomyelitis and abscess. AJR Am J Roentgenol 2002;178:215–22.
[20] Enderle MD, Coerper S, Schweizer HP, et al. Correlation of imaging techniques to histopathology in patients with diabetic foot syndrome and clinical suspecion of chronic osteomyelitis. The role of high-resolution ultrasound. Diabetes Care 1999;22:294–9.
[21] O'Meara SM, Cullum NA, Majid M, Sheldon TA. Systemic review of antimicrobial agents used for chronic wounds. Br J Surg 2001;88:4–21.
[22] Lipsky BA. Evidence-based antibiotic therapy of diabetic foot infections. FEMS Immunol Med Microbiol 1999;26:267–76.
[23] Armstrong DG, Findlow AH, Oyibo SO, Boulton AJM. The use of absorbable antibiotic-impregnated calcium sulphate pellets in the management of diabetic foot infections. Diabet Med 2001; 11:942.
[24] Nuermberger E, Auwaerter P. Johns Hopkins Division of Infectious Disease Antibiotic Guide. Baltimore (MD): Johns Hopkins University Division of Infectious Disease; 2002. Available at: abxfeedback@hopkins-abxguide.org.
[25] Nix DE, Cumbo TJ, Kuritzsky P, et al. Oral ciprofloxacin in the treatment of serious soft tissue and bone infection: efficacy, safety, and pharmokinetics. Am J Med 1987;82:146–53.
[26] Lipsky BA, Baker PD, Landon GC, Fernau R. Antibiotic therapy for diabetic foot infections: comparison of two parenteral-to-oral regimens. Clin Infect Dis 1997;24:643–8.
[27] Sesin GP, Paszko A, O'Keefe E. Oral clindamycin and ciprofloxacin therapy for diabetic foot infections. Pharmacotherapy 1990;10:154–6.
[28] Goldstein EJ, Citron DM, Nesbit CA. Diabetic foot infections. Bacteriology and activity of 10 oral antimicrobial agents against bacteria isolated from consecutive cases. Diabetes Care 1996;19: 638–41.
[29] Siami G, Christou N, Eiseman I, Tack KJ. Clinafloxacin versus pipercillin-tazobactam in treatment of patients with severe skin and soft tissue infections. Antimicrob Agents Chemother 2001;45: 525–31.

[30] Senneville E, Yazdanpanah Y, Cazaubiel M, et al. Rifampicin-ofloxacin oral regimen for the treatment of mild to moderate diabetic foot osteomyelitis. J Antimicrob Chemother 2001;48:927–30.
[31] Rissing JP. Antimicrobial therapy for chronic osteomyelitis in adults: role of the quinolones. Clin Infect Dis 1997;25:1327–33.
[32] Zurenko GE, Yagi BH, Schaadt RD, et al. In vitro activities of U-100592 and U-100766, novel oxazolidinone antibacterial agents. Antimicrob Agents Chemother 1996;40:839–45.
[33] Miyasaki S, Fujikawa T, Kobayashi I, et al. The in vitro and in vivo antibacterial characterization of vancomycin and linezolid against vancomycin-susceptible and resistant enterococci. J Antimicrob Chemother 2002;50:971–4.
[34] Rubinstein E, Cammarata SK, Oliphant TH, et al, and the Linezolid Nosocomial Pneumonia Study Group. Linezolid PNU-100766) versus vancomycin in the treatment of hospitalized patients with nosocomial pneumonia: a randomized, double-blind, multicenter study. Clin Infect Dis 2001; 32:402–12.
[35] Stevens DL, Herr D, Lampiris H, et al, and the Linezolid MRSA Study Group. Linezolid versus vancomycin for the treatment of methicillin-resistant Staphylococcus aureus infections. Clin Infect Dis 2002;34:1481–90.
[36] Tentolouris N, Jude EB, Smirnof I, et al. Methicillin-resistant staphylococcus aureus: an increasing problem in a diabetic foot clinic. Diabet Med 1999;16:767–71.
[37] Roghmann MC, Siddiqui A, Plaisance K, Standiford H. MRSA colonization and the risk of MRSA bacteraemia in hospitalized patients with chronic ulcers. J Hosp Infect 2001;47:98–103.
[38] Dang CN, Prasad YDM, Boulton AJM, Jude EB. Methicillin-resistant Staphylococcus aureus in the diabetic foot clinic: a worsening problem. Diabet Med 2003;20:159–61.
[39] Lautenbach E, LaRosa LA, Marr AM, et al. Changes in the prevalence of vancomycin-resistant enterococci in response to antimicrobial formulary interventions: impact of progressive restrictions on use of vancomycin and third-generation cephalosporins. Clin Infect Dis 2003;36:440–6.
[40] Lipsky BA. Osteomyelitis of the foot in diabetic patients. Clin Infect Dis 1997;25:1318–26.
[41] Venkatesan P, Lawn S, Macfarlane RM, et al. Conservative management of osteomyelitis in the feet of diabetic patients. Diabet Med 1997;14:487–90.
[42] Klepser ME, Marangos MN, Zhu Z, et al. Comparison of the bactericidal activities of piperacillin-tazobactam, ticarciliin-clavulanate, and ampicillin-sulbactam against clinical isolates of Bacteroides fragilis, Enterococcus faecalis, Escherichia coli, and Pseudomonas aeruginosa. Antimicrob Agents Chemother 1997;41:435–9.
[43] Zeillemaker AM, Veldkamp KE, Van Kraaij MG, et al. Pipercillin/tazobactam therapy for diabetic foot infection. Foot Ankle Int 1998;19:169–72.
[44] File TM, Tan JS. Ticarcillin-clavulanate therapy for bacterial skin and soft tissue infections. Rev Infect Dis 1991;13:733–6.
[45] Akova M, Ozcebe O, Gullu I, et al. Efficacy of sulbactam-ampicillin for the treatment of severe diabetic foot infections. J Chemother 1996;8:284–9.
[46] Raymakers JT, Houben AJ, Heyden JJ, et al. The effect of diabetes and severe ischaemia on the penetration of ceftazidime into tissue of the limb. Diabet Med 2001;18:229–34.
[47] Grayson ML, Gibbons GW, Habershaw GM, et al. Use of ampicillin/sulbactam versus imipenem/cilastin in the treatment of limb-threatening foot infections in diabetic patients. Clin Infect Dis 1994;18:683–93.
[48] Pathare NA, Sathe SR. Antibiotic combinations in polymicrobic diabetic foot infections. Indian J Med Sci 2001;12:655–62.
[49] Diamantopoulos EJ, Haritos D, Yfandi G, et al. Management and outcome of severe diabetic foot infections. Exp Clin Endocrinol Diabetes 1998;106:346–52.
[50] Seabrook GR, Edmiston CE, Schmitt DD, et al. Comparison of serum and tissue antibiotic levels in diabetes-related foot infections. Surgery 1991;110:671.
[51] Nehler MR, Whitehill TA, Bowers SP, et al. Intermediate-term outcome of primary digit amputation in patients with diabetes mellitus who have forefoot sepsis requiring hospitalization and presumed adequate circulatory status. J Vasc Surg 1999;30:509–17.
[52] Bamberger DM, Duas GP, Gerding DN. Osteomyelitis in the feet of diabetic patients: long-term

results, prognostic factors, and the role of antimicrobial and surgical therapy. Am J Med 1987;83: 653–60.
[53] Lipsky BA, Pecoraro RE, Larson SA, et al. Outpatient management of uncomplicated lower-extremity infections in diabetic patients. Arch Intern Med 1990;150:790–7.
[54] Bertoni AG, Saydah S, Brancati FL. Diabetes and the risk of infection-related mortality in the US. Diabetes Care 2001;24:1044–9.
[55] Eckmam MH, Greenfield S, Mackey WC, et al. Foot infections in diabetic patients: decision and cost-effectiveness analysis. JAMA 1995;273:712–20.

Clin Podiatr Med Surg
20 (2003) 671–688

CLINICS IN PODIATRIC MEDICINE AND SURGERY

Medical evaluation and treatment of diabetic peripheral neuropathy

William A. Petit, Jr, MD, FACP, FACE*,
Raghu P. Upender, MD

The Joslin Clinic for Diabetes, New Britain General Hospital, 100 Grand Street, New Britain, CT 06050, USA

Diabetes is one of the major public health concerns facing the modern world. If current trends prevail, the number of people afflicted by diabetes worldwide will double by 2025 to almost 300 million [1]. Ironically, it is human success that is contributing to the rise in the incidence of diabetes. First, agricultural success has led to increased access to food, which has encouraged overeating and obesity, a well-recognized risk factor for diabetes. Second, increased automation at work and proliferation of motorized transportation has led to lifestyles that are increasingly sedentary. Physical exercise, which is known to protect against diabetes, is limited or lacking for many individuals. Last, medical advances in prolonging lives have led to an ever aging population. Because diabetes is still predominantly a disease of middle and later years, it is not surprising that its prevalence is increasing as the population ages.

The morbidity and mortality of diabetes is related to the development of macrovascular and microvascular complications. Macrovascular complications include myocardial ischemia, stroke, and peripheral vascular disease. Microvascular injury resulting from chronic hyperglycemia causes retinopathy, nephropathy, and neuropathy. The combination of peripheral vascular disease and neuropathy leads to one of the most feared diabetic complications, the diabetic foot, which is the leading cause of nontraumatic limb amputation in the United States [2]. The impact of diabetic foot complications on the individual and society is enormous. The immobility, loss of independence, and frequent hospitalizations severely diminish these patients' quality of life. The direct and indirect annual cost to society is also immense. In Geneva, Switzerland, the cost of nine below-knee amputations is estimated to be equal to the annual salary of a clinical team of three doctors, five nurses, one dietitian, three auxiliary staff, and one secretary [1]. Because treatments

* Corresponding author.
E-mail address: docp@cox.net (W.A. Petit, Jr).

doi:10.1016/S0891-8422(03)00068-5

options are limited, and frequently unsatisfactory, prevention of diabetic foot complications becomes even more imperative. Prevention begins with the early identification of risk factors. One of the most important risk factors for the diabetic foot is diabetic neuropathy. This article reviews our current understanding of diabetic neuropathy.

Epidemiology

Diabetic neuropathy is defined as "peripheral, somatic or autonomic nerve damage attributable solely to diabetes mellitus" [3]. The measures used to determine the presence of neuropathy vary greatly between published studies; consequently, the reported prevalence of neuropathy in diabetic patients ranges from 5% to 80%. A recent National Health Interview survey questioned a large representative sample of US adults about symptoms of sensory neuropathy that included numbness, pain, tingling, and altered temperature sensation in the hands or feet [4]. Among those with self-reported diabetes, 37.9% had one or more of these symptoms, compared with only about 10% of the population without diabetes. The Pittsburgh Epidemiology of Diabetes Complications Study estimated the prevalence of diabetic polyneuropathy (defined as symptoms consistent with neuropathy, presence of two or more sensory or motor signs, and decreased tendon reflexes) in patients with type 1 diabetes older than 30 at 58% [5]. Using comprehensive measures of neuropathy that included symptoms, signs, nerve conduction studies, quantitative sensory testing, and autonomic testing, the Rochester Diabetic Neuropathy study reported a prevalence of 60.8% [6,7]. European estimates of prevalence are somewhat lower. A large cross-sectional study of 6487 diabetic patients in the United Kingdom found the prevalence of diabetic neuropathy to be 28.5% [8]. Among residents of East Dorset, England, the prevalence of diabetic neuropathy was 13% for type 1 diabetes and 17% for patients with type 2 diabetes [9]. In the Piemonte region of Italy, 28% of 467 individuals with type 1 diabetes had neuropathy as defined by abnormalities on a structured questionnaire, objective neurological evaluation, and autonomic testing [10]. In rural Australia, the prevalence of neuropathy in patients with type 1 diabetes was only 8% [11].

Epidemiological studies have also assessed risk factors for diabetic neuropathy. It is well recognized that the risk of developing neuropathy increases with the duration of diabetes [12]. Pirart found that the prevalence of neuropathy rose from about 8% at the time of diagnosis to about 50% 25 years later in his cohort of 2795 patients who have diabetes and who were followed from the onset of their disease [13,14]. In the National Health Interview Survey of 2392 patients who self-reported diabetes, the independent risk factors for sensory neuropathy were increasing duration of diabetes, hypertension, and high blood glucose [4]. The Pittsburgh Epidemiology of Diabetes Complications Study identified increasing duration of diabetes, elevated glycosylated hemoglobin (HbA1c), lower high-density lipoprotein levels, cigarette smoking, and the presence of overt nephropathy or proliferative retinopathy as independent predictors of neuropathy

[5]. In the Diabetes Control and Complications Trial, those who had neuropathy were older and were more likely to be men, taller, have retinopathy, and have had a longer duration of disease [15]. Increasing age and longer duration of diabetes were risk factors for diabetic neuropathy in the Piemonte study [10]. Height and retinopathy were independent predictors of neuropathy among patients with type 1 DM in East Dorset, England [9].

Classification

Diabetes affects the peripheral nerve at various sites and can lead to mononeuropathy, polyneuropathy, plexopathy, and radiculopathy. Clinically, it is important to distinguish between symmetric and asymmetric neuropathies because they differ in pathologic mechanisms and require different diagnostic and therapeutic approaches. The most common neuropathy in diabetes is diabetic polyneuropathy (DPN), a symmetric length-dependent sensorimotor neuropathy. Sensory symptoms predominate early in DPN because sensory fibers are longer and more vulnerable to metabolic-microvascular damage. Sensory ataxia and motor weakness develops later. There is variability in the presentation of DPN. Some patients experience severe neuropathic pain without much motor weakness or numbness, suggesting involvement of small sensory fibers, whereas others are unaware of neuropathy until significant weakness and gait disturbance develops, implicating larger sensory-motor fiber dysfunction. Although this dichotomy between small and large fiber neuropathy is clinically accepted, it is not supported by pathologic studies. Dyck and associates postulate that the so-called "variants of DPN" may actually be extremes of a normal distribution of DPN. Studying sural nerve biopsies, they found that the ratio of small to large myelinated fibers were more variable in DPN patients than in controls, but no clustering of cases with large or small fiber loss was seen [16]. Autonomic neuropathy is included with distal symmetrical sensory polyneuropathies because the results of thermoregulatory sweat testing in most patients with autonomic neuropathy demonstrate a length-dependent loss of sweating [17].

Rarely will patients who have diabetes develop the syndrome consisting of a subacute onset and progressive distal and proximal symmetric motor neuropathy with increased protein in cerebrospinal fluid (albumino-cytologic disassociation). The presentation, course and response to immunomodulating therapy are similar to chronic inflammatory demyelinating polyradiculoneuropathy (CIDP).

Of the asymmetric diabetic neuropathies, diabetic lumbosacral radiculoplexus neuropathy (DLSRPN) is the most distinct disorder. It is also known as diabetic amyotrophy, proximal diabetic neuropathy, and femoral neuropathy. It occurs as a monophasic illness during periods of poor glycemic control and significant weight loss. DLSRPN affects mostly men with type 2 diabetes and is thought to be associated with an inflammatory angiopathy. Typically, patients experience subacute onset of unilateral hip and thigh pain that can last for days. Before the pain resolves, patients develop weakness of their hip flexors and adductors, and most prominently knee extensors. Recovery is slow and can take 6 to 24 months. Incomplete recoveries are not uncommon. A related condition known as diabetic thoracolumbar radiculopathy presents mainly with radicular pain and numbness [18].

Isolated cranial neuropathies are not rare in patients who have type 1 and type 2 diabetes. Cranial nerves three, four, six, and seven are the most commonly affected nerves. The typical presentation of diabetic oculomotor palsy is acute onset ipsilateral headache, diplopia, ptosis, and spared papillary function [19]. Cranial neuropathies can occur in the presence or absence of DPN and, therefore, they probably do not share the same pathologic mechanism. Histopathological studies support a mechanism of focal ischemia resulting in segmental demyelination and remyelination. Similar vascular mechanisms may be involved in the rare condition mononeuritis multiplex, which can occur in conjunction with diabetic polyneuropathy.

Other asymmetric neuropathies are caused by nerve compression and repetitive nerve injury. These include median neuropathy at the wrist (carpal tunnel syndrome), ulnar neuropathy at the elbow (cubital tunnel syndrome), lateral femoral cutaneous sensory neuropathy (meralgia paresthetica), and tibial neuropathy at the ankle (tarsal tunnel syndrome).

Clinical course of diabetic polyneuropathy

In type 1 and type 2 diabetes mellitus, diabetic polyneuropathy usually develops after many years of hyperglycemia. Because the exact time of onset of type 2 diabetes mellitus is not always obvious in some patients, DPN can be present at the time of diagnosis (presumably because of the unrecognized chronic hyperglycemia). Diabetic polyneuropathy begins with abnormal nerve conduction or abnormality of heart rate variability during deep breathing. As the neuropathy progresses, ankle reflexes are lost; vibration perception is reduced; and, eventually, frank sensory loss becomes apparent. DPN is a length-dependent process that is sometimes described as "dying back" neuropathy. Sensory fibers, which are typically the longest, become affected early and lead to abnormal sensations. Patients describe "numb" or "dead" sensations as well as tightness, and prickling sensations. Some patients experience prominent burning pain with or without numbness. As neuropathy progresses, more proximal motor fibers become affected and lead to distal limb weakness. Involvement of sensory and motor fibers eventually leads to gait impairment. The presence of uremia and poor glycemic control (hyper- and hypoglycemia) often leads to more severe manifestations of neuropathy. Autonomic symptoms, such as gastroparesis, erectile dysfunction, diarrhea, and sphincter dysfunction, may occur at any stage of the neuropathy and will be disabling [17].

Diagnosis

Diagnosis of neuropathy is not difficult when a patient presents with typical symptoms of symmetric distal lower limb numbness or pain. The challenge for the health care professional lies in the early detection of neuropathy, even before patients are themselves aware. Early recognition of neuropathy will lead to greater vigilance for one of the feared complications of diabetic polyneuropathy, the diabetic foot. Early recognition of neuropathy may lead to real efforts in risk modification, including more prudent glycemic control, the only intervention affecting the course of DPN. Several screening tools have been developed, and with their aid early detection of neuropathy is possible [20–22]. These screening tools typically employ simple questionnaires and an abridged neurological exam. They are quick, easy to use, and provide high sensitivity if not specificity. More comprehensive neuropathy tests have been developed to quantify neuropathy symptoms and signs. They are used mainly as research tools. These include neuropathy symptoms score (NSS), neuropathy impairment score (NIS), and neuropathy symptoms profile (NSP) [23–25]. Use of the Semmes-Weinstein monofilament offers a simple, standardized, quick, and inexpensive bedside test for the presence of neuropathy. This screening test identifies those at most risk of developing diabetic foot ulcers due to loss of sensation. A more detailed neurological exam that includes tests of various sensory modalities (vibration, nociception, proprioception, and light touch), muscle stretch reflexes, motor strength, and gait stability allows more complete assessment of the functional integrity of the peripheral nervous system.

Electrophysiologic studies are also helpful in early detection of neuropathy. As mentioned above, the earliest manifestation of DPN is slowing of nerve conduction [26]. Nerve conduction studies (NCS) are minimally invasive tests that are widely available and standardized. In addition to confirming and quantifying nerve dysfunction, NCS are useful in elucidating the pathologic features of neuropathy, such as demyelination and axonal loss. Nerve conduction studies are performed by stimulating a nerve at various proximal sites while recording from either the muscle for motor nerves or distal nerve branch for sensory nerves. Needle electromyography is often performed in conjunction with NCS and provides further evaluation of the motor nerve function.

Quantitative sensory testing (QST) is another way of detecting and quantifying DPN. Dyck and associates [27] first introduced automated quantitative sensory testing in 1975. The computer-assisted sensory examination (CASE) IV system uses physiologic stimuli to quantify sensory nerve dysfunction. Comparing the thresholds at which a patient detects a particular stimulus with normative data provides a percentile score of sensory loss that can be followed over time. Vibration detection threshold and heat and cold detection have been standardized. The presence of autonomic neuropathy can be evaluated by measuring heart rate variation with deep breathing. Sudomotor function has been evaluated with quantitative sudomotor axon reflex test (Q-SART). Using the above quantitative neuropathy tests, diabetic neuropathy can be staged. Staging is clinically useful and provides the patient and the health care provider a cumulative measure that can be followed clinically as the neuropathy progresses [24].

Once the neuropathy is identified, the next challenge is distinguishing DPN from other varieties of sensorimotor polyneuropathy, such as inherited, immune (Sjogren's syndrome), toxic (alcohol, medicinal), metabolic (uremia, hepatic, and others), and malnutrition. The distinction between etiologies is crucial to the appropriate management of neuropathy. Neuropathy in patients who have is not always due to diabetes. In one study, up to 20% of patients diagnosed with diabetic polyneuropathy were found to have other etiologies causing the neuropathy [28]. Diabetic polyneuropathy often occurs in association with diabetic retinopathy or nephropathy. The absence of either of these complications makes the diagnosis of DPN questionable. Review of medical history with specific attention to family history, occupational exposures, personal habits, and medication exposure usually helps exclude many of the less common causes of neuropathy. Physical exam helps identify atypical patterns of sensory loss or weakness that may suggest an alternative diagnosis. Electrophysiologic studies help exclude demyelinating neuropathies. Routine blood work helps identify metabolic derangements, endocrinopathies, paraproteinemia, vitamin deficiencies, heavy metal exposure, and collagen vascular diseases. Less common blood tests help identify autoantibodies reactive against peripheral nerve epitopes. Nerve and muscle biopsy may provide further clues to the etiology of the neuropathy. Nerve biopsies are most useful in diagnosing inflammatory neuropathy, such as perineuritis and peripheral nerve vasculitisc. Not every patient who has diabetes needs extensive and often expensive laboratory evaluation. The extent of evaluation should be guided by the severity and functional consequences of the neuropathy.

Pathology

As discussed above, diabetic neuropathy can become manifest in varied ways and therefore it is not surprising that different pathologic mechanisms are involved in various types of diabetic neuropathy. Currently, at least four mechanisms are implicated: metabolic-microvascular derangement (hyperglycemic), immune, compression, and hypoglycemia [26,29]. In diabetic polyneuropathy (DPN), metabolic-microvascular derangement may be the most important mechanism. Other microvascular complications of diabetes, such as retinopathy and nephropathy, are statistically associated with DPN, suggesting these complications share similar pathologic mechanisms. Under an electron microscope, various structural abnormalities can be seen within the endoneurium of diabetic nerves, including endothelial cell hyperplasia [30], capillary closure [23], thrombosis [31], thickening of or reduplication of capillary wall basement membranes [32], endothelial and pericyte degeneration [33], and endothelial fenestration and dysjunction [34]. The degree of microvascular derangements appears to correlate with the severity of DPN. Various nerve fiber abnormalities have been reported in diabetic polyneuropathy, including axonal degeneration, regeneration, and segmental demyelination and remyelination [26].

Although several lines of evidence link microvascular derangements to DPN, it is not clear whether chronic hyperglycemia leads directly to nerve fiber injury (axonal or neuronal and Schwann cells) or microvascular injury first and then nerve fiber injury secondarily. Animal and in vitro experiments over the past 25 years point to oxidative stress as the underlying cause of microvascular damage and nerve fiber injury. Four major pathways of glucose metabolism are implicated in the development of microvascular complications. These include (1) activation of polyol pathway; (2) activation of protein kinase C (PKC); (3) accumulation of advanced glycation end products [35]; and (4) increased hexosamine pathway flux [36]. Hyperglycemia causes perturbation of each of these pathways directly or indirectly and leads to overproduction of superoxides that leads to tissue damage.

Chronically elevated blood glucose leads to activation of the polyol pathway that leads to sorbitol and fructose accumulation, NAD(P)H-redox imbalance, and increase in PKC activity. Increased protein kinase C activity leads to altered vascular permeability, contractility, basement membrane synthesis, and cellular proliferation, all of which may lead to the development of diabetic microvascular complications [37]. Supporting this notion, the PKC inhibitor, LY333531, appears to decrease vascular endothelial growth factor (VEGF) and thereby inhibit intraocular neovascularization caused by retinal ischemia [38,39]. A large, double-blind, placebo-controlled, randomized, multicenter trial of LY333531 in diabetic polyneuropathy is currently underway.

Hyperglycemia leads to nonenzymatic glycation of proteins that then cross-link to form advanced glycation end products (AGEs). The cross-linking of these proteins alters their structure and function. This may account for the observed slowing of axonal transport in DPN. Hyperglycemia also leads to impaired phospholipid and fatty acid metabolism. Linoleic acid conversion to γ-linolenic acid (GLA) is impaired in diabetes. This results in the altered metabolisms of prostaglandinds that in turn leads to nerve dysfunction. In a double-blind, placebo-controlled, randomized, multicenter study, peroneal and median motor NCV and thermal perception threshold improved in the patients randomized to evening primrose oil (GLA) treatment compared with the control patients [40]. The confluence of these various metabolic and vascular disturbances leads to impaired neural function and loss of neurotrophic support and, over time, can mediate apoptosis of neurons and Schwann cells.

Medical management of diabetic polyneuropathy

Glycemic control

Despite the many advances in the treatment of type 1 and type 2 diabetes mellitus over the past 80 years, including insulin, sulfonylureas, thiazolidinediones, insulin pumps, laser therapy, angiotensin-converting enzyme inhibitors/angiotensin receptor blockers, and HMG-Co A reductase inhibitors, there has been no breakthrough—no true blockbuster therapy—for the treatment of diabetic neuropathy. The first therapy for all patients who have any microvascular or metabolic complication of type 1 or type 2 diabetes mellitus is attempting to normalize blood glucose levels. This is not directly within the purview of the podiatrist or orthopedic surgeon, but it is critical for all members of the diabetes care team to reinforce this notion with all patients seeking care for painful neuropathic syndromes. The Diabetes Control and Complications Trial (DCCT) and the United Kingdom Prospective Diabetes Study (UKPDS) showed that improved glycemic control would lessen the risk of developing neuropathy in patients who have type 1 and type 2 diabetes. They also showed that there would be less progression of neuropathy in those who already had the complication (mainly in the UKPDS as most patients in the DCCT had no neuropathy at the time of entry into the trial). There was a 71% decrease in the development of new neuropathy in the tightly controlled (Hgb A1C = 7.0%) primary prevention cohort of patients in the DCCT (9.6% new neuropathy in the standard group versus 2.8% in the experimental group) [15,41]. In the secondary intervention group the reduction was 64% (6.7% versus 16.9%). In the UKPDS, more patients in the standard therapy group progressed to a sensory endpoint that put them at greater risk of ulcer development than the intensively treated group [42].

Significant changes in glycemic control can lead to acute sensory symptoms. These symptoms will often respond to improvements in blood glucose levels. This acute neuropathy or neuritis may be partly metabolic and partly vascular as a result of perineural ischemia. Many clinicians have advised rapidly controlling glucose levels with intravenous or continuous subcutaneous insulin infusions. When a patient improves glycemic control there is often a tingling or dysesthetic sensation, which may be caused by changes in the vasa nervorum or nerve regeneration [20,43,44]. Improved glycemic control leads to decreased sorbitol uptake into nerve, improved intracellular myoinositol levels, better neural bioenergetics, improved endothelial function, and better blood flow in the vasa nervorum. Improved glycemic control has also been found to decrease production of advanced glycosylation end products [33,45,46].

Attempts to find therapies that affect the natural course of diabetic neuropathy have been unsuccessful to date. A multicenter trial on the efficacy of recombinant human nerve growth failed to show any discernible clinical benefit in the 1019 patients who participated [47]. Aldose reductase inhibitors have been studied for a number of years based on sorbitol's metabolic role in DPN. Unfortunately, multiple trials have shown either inconsistent results or serious adverse effects. Thus none are yet clinically available for use in the United States [48]. Because oxidative stress is believed to be part of all the complications of diabetes, many investigators are now looking at a number of vitamins and herbs to diminish direct oxidative damage to the nerve or the vasa nervorum. To date, the published trial shows a small improvement in neuropathic symptoms but little effect chronically [49,50].

Treatment of pain

Because therapies affecting the natural course of diabetic neuropathy are limited, treatment strategies have focused on symptom control. Many patients who have neuropathy suffer from chronic intractable pain. Over the past 38 years, we have learned much about the transmission of pain by way of A delta and C fibers. These myelinated and unmyelinated nerves transmit painful stimuli to the dorsal horn, spinothalamic tracts, thalamus, and sensory cortex. Investigation into the peripheral and central pain pathways has led to the identification of the neurotransmitters involved pain transmission. Thus medications aimed at substance P, N-methyl-D-aspartate (NMDA), glutamate, membrane stabilization, mitogen-activated protein kinases, and cytokines have been more clinically helpful.

Simple analgesics

For mild symptoms it is reasonable to begin with acetaminophen. Though some patients have tried it before their office visit, many have not and if they have, it is usually at subtherapeutic dosages. We typically advise patients to use an extended-relief acetaminophen preparation that provides 650 to 1300 mg in a dose. Most patients have their most debilitating and annoying symptoms at bedtime and may only need to be dosed at that time. Many patients complain of a hyperesthetic sensation to the bedclothes and some will actually respond by wearing stockings or soft slippers to bed. Presumably this helps because, according to the gate control theory of Melzack and Wall [51], stimulation of the A-beta fibers that transmit proprioception and pressure signals overrides painful sensory signals from the smaller C fibers. In some patients whose symptoms increase at night, any mild hypnotic that allows them to fall asleep may diminish pain. Diphenhydramine (25–50 mg), melatonin (1–3 mg), zolpidem (5–10 mg), and small doses of benzodiazepines (variable) may be helpful, though those in the last group of medications are potentially addictive [52].

Other nonnarcotic analgesics have limited use. We try to avoid nonsteroidal anti-inflammatory drugs in diabetic patients because they decrease prostacyclin levels, which in turn lead to decreased renal blood flow and worsening of renal function, fluid retention, and possible exacerbation of any underlying hypertension and congestive heart failure. Cohen and Harris published data [53] from a small group of patients at a Veterans Administration hospital noting diminished pain with 2400 mg of ibuprofen or 400 mg of sulindac daily. This is consistent with our clinical experience of patients who have mild to moderate symptoms who are able to tolerate these agents. There is currently no good published data on the newer COX-II antagonists.

Opioids and other analgesics

The use of narcotics in the treatment of painful sensory neuropathy is controversial because of their long-term complications, especially in the elderly. These agents may decrease cognitive function, which can worsen the perception of hypoglycemia. Narcotics can lead to severe constipation by slowing gut motility in patients who may already be suffering from autonomic neuropathy. These factors, along with the risk of tolerance and addiction, further limit their use. Despite these potential problems, there are patients who have severe and disabling neuropathic pain who respond only to narcotic analgesics. A recent study of the long-acting form of oxycodone has been completed, but the results have not yet been published. The authors typically use the lowest dose of a narcotic for the shortest period of time, though many of these patients require chronic dosing. We see less adverse effects with oxycodone and hydrocodone compared with codeine, and meperidine and hydromorphone have inadequate half-lives to be useful chronically. Patients using these agents must typically be a on a bowel regiment with senna or docusate or polyethylene glycol with cathartics used every 2 to 4 days as needed to avoid severe constipation.

Tramadol (classified differently than the NSAIDs and the narcotics) improved sleep and pain in a double-blind randomized trial of 131 patients and an open-label extension. The dropout rate was nearly 15% [54,55]. We have seen similar results in our patients and find tramadol safe and usually nonaddicting. Starting at a low dose of 50 mg at bedtime seems to help patients avoid the dizziness, nausea, and other CNS symptoms that typically occur early on and then fade. Typically doses of 50 to 100 mg (daily maximum 400 mg) dosed every 6 hours are necessary.

Antidepressant medications

Tricyclic antidepressant (TCA) drugs have been the mainstays of symptomatic neuropathy therapy for many years because they directly impact sensory symptoms and can also treat depressive and anxiety complaints. In addition, the anticholinergic sedative properties of these agents have been used to help patients sleep. Presumably these drugs work by decreasing the uptake of serotonin and norepinephrine at the nerve synapse. They may also have an effect on the alpha-1 adrenergic receptors and sympathetic activity. Much of the data has been obtained with amitriptyline and imipramine. Their adverse effects, namely, the previously mentioned sedation, blurred vision (changes in ability to accommodate, more common in older patients), dry mouth, and diminished ability to urinate (much more common in older men) have limited the usefulness of these drugs. More serious side effects, such as arrhythmias and orthostatic hypotension, must be considered as these agents are often used in older patients who have concomitant cardiac dysfunction. Fortunately, these drugs often work at fairly low dosages, typically at lower doses than is needed to achieve antidepressant effects. By starting at a low dose and slowly increasing it, side effects may be minimized. In an early trial of imipramine, 12 patients who have painful neuropathy were studied in a fixed-dose, crossover, double-blind trial. Seven of 12 had decreased pain, numbness, dysesthesias, and nocturnal worsening versus 0 of 12 on the placebo [56]. Because amitriptyline is metabolized to nortriptyline and seems to have fewer side effects, many patients are begun on nortriptyline, 10 to 25 mg at bedtime, or on imipramine, 25 to 50 mg. Often the dosage must be increased to 100 to 150 mg/d for amitriptyline, nortriptyline, and imipramine, or desipramine, though most studies have not shown a good relationship of symptom relief to dosage or plasma levels. However, when starting slowly it takes a much longer time to achieve a therapeutic effect. In a study of amitriptyline, desipramine, and fluoxetine, the first two drugs were superior to placebo in relief of pain and worked in depressed and nondepressed patients. The authors noted that patients better tolerated desipramine; tricyclic antidepressants and their preferential blockade of norepinephrine reuptake appear to be more effective. Unfortunately, the serotonin-specific reuptake inhibitor fluoxetine, though much better tolerated, was no better than placebo, again indicating that the adrenergic effect was crucial [57]. In a much earlier article, amitriptyline was combined with fluphenazine and pain relief was seen quickly, within the first week. This study was limited by the fact that only eight patients were studied [58]. There has been one article suggesting that the SSRI drug paroxetine might also be beneficial. It was compared with imipramine in a randomized double-blind, crossover study using 40 mg of paroxetine and a variable dose of imipramine. Paroxetine reduced observer-noted and self-reported symptoms but was slightly less effective than the imipramine. However, the paroxetine was better tolerated and caused less dropouts and no withdrawal symptoms as the imipramine did [59]. There have been a number of reports that venlafaxine, another serotonin and norepinephrine reuptake inhibitor, may be useful as an analgesic in the treatment of painful neuropathy. It can cause some nausea, dizziness, and sleepiness, but is well tolerated and available as an extended relief capsule [60–62].

Anticonvulsants

Phenytoin has been recommended and used for years to treat painful diabetic neuropathy, much of the interest based on case reports from the 1940s through the 1960s. However, the controlled studies with phenytoin were unable to show any efficacy and at this time this drug cannot be recommended [63,64].

Carbamazepine has been successfully used in patients who have a lancinating quality to their neuropathic pain. It can be effective at fairly low doses, but because of possible significant side effects (leukopenia and hepatotoxicity), it should be used after safer drugs have been tried and failed. Patients must have complete blood counts and liver function test monitoring to avoid serious side effects. The oldest reference is a small double-blind trial that showed a small improvement in symptoms in patients who have mild neuropathy [65]. Other small trials have also shown positive effects on symptoms and nerve conduction [22,66,67].

Currently the most widely used agent outside of the TCA drugs is gabapentin (formally FDA approved for the treatment of complex partial seizures). It is structurally similar to gamma-aminobutyric acid (GABA), which is a neurotransmitter involved in the transmission and modulation of pain signals. It appears to work by way of sodium and calcium channels at the level of the spinal cord. There have been at least two large controlled trails using gabapentin, and both have been positive. One study was a multicenter, double-blind, randomized, placebo-controlled trial of 165 patients, 84 of which received gabapentin. Eighty-three percent of the patients completed the 8-week trial. Dosages ranged from 900 to 3600 mg/d. Using an intent-to-treat analysis, the gabapentin-treated patients had significantly lower pain scores ($P < 0.001$). Quality-of-life scores were also higher in the active treatment group. Dizziness and sleepiness were the most common side effects seen but did not cause excessive dropouts. There was also slightly more confusion in the gabapentin group (8% versus 1.2%, $P = 0.06$). Despite this, the quality-of-life scores were universally higher in the gabapentin-treated group [68]. In another study, which compared gabapentin (mean dose 1565 mg) and amitriptyline (mean dose 59 mg), improvements in pain score were shown with both drugs, but neither was superior to the other. Twenty-one of 25 patients completed the trial. The amitriptyline caused more side effects and more weight gain compared with the gabapentin [69].

Lamotrigine is an anticonvulsant that works by way of the sodium channel and also blocks presynaptic glutamate receptors. Several small and short-term trials using 200 to 400 mg/d of lamotrigine have shown decreases in pain versus placebo, and side effects were similar in both groups [70,71].

Topiramate is another anticonvulsant that has been recently been used for the treatment of painful diabetic neuropathy and has caused some excitement because of its potential effect of helping with weight loss. It appears to work by way of sodium channels and by accentuating GABA activity. However, most studies to date have not shown decreases in pain. In addition, slow titration is required to avoid cognitive side effects [25].

Antiarrhythmic agents

Lidocaine is an antiarrhythmic agent available for intravenous use. Patients treated with lidocaine require continuous electrocardiographic monitoring and thus this agent has been mainly used in desperate cases where all oral and outpatient therapies have failed. There are data to show short-term efficacy [72].

Mexiletine is a class IIb antiarrhythmic and an oral analog of lidocaine. There are four studies in the literature, two of which show mexiletine to be superior to placebo. Dosages used have varied widely from 200 to 700 mg [45,73–75]. This drug is potentially proarrhythmic. A major concern is that by clinical definition all patients who have diabetes are in a secondary cardiac prevention category. These two issues have caused most physicians to be cautious in using this drug. Many will not use it without cardiology clearance or initial in-patient monitoring. The 1988 report on 16 patients completing a randomized double-blind crossover trial of mexiletine (10 mg/kg/d) showed a significant decrease in pain using a visual analog scale versus placebo. There were no changes in beat-to-beat variation in the treated patients and no significant arrhythmias [45]. Two-hundred sixteen insulin-treated patients who have diabetes were treated with dosages up to 675 mg/d and showed diminished pain, as measured by the visual analog scale, and improved sleep. Twenty-four hour electrocardiographic mapping did not reveal any significant arrhythmias [73]. For small areas of neuropathic pain the use of the topical lidocaine patch has been helpful with little or no toxicity. Most of the efficacy data with this therapy has been generated in the treatment of postherpetic neuralgia.

Topical therapies

Capsaicin is the active ingredient in hot peppers and will deplete substance P from nerve tissue and decrease pain. Practically, there have been two issues: (1) unless it is homemade (1–4 teaspoons of Cayenne pepper in a 4-ounce jar of cold cream and applied with disposable gloves) or the area being treated is small, the cost can be high; and (2) there is often an increase in burning or a form of hyperesthesia that occurs for the first 2 weeks as the capsaicin is applied. Often patients are unable to tolerate this and stop therapy before any benefit is gained. In a multicenter trial involving 277 patients treated over an 8-week period using a double-blind vehicle-controlled design versus 0.075% capsaicin cream, pain decreased and activities of daily living as well as quality of life improved for the patients on active therapy [76]. A meta-analysis also concurred that capsaicin was effective as therapy [77].

Other medications/therapies

Amantadine therapy was used in a recent pilot study of 17 patients who have painful diabetic neuropathy. It was considered for use because amantadine is a noncompetitive antagonist of the N-methyl-D-aspartate excitatory receptor involved in nociceptive signaling. Amantadine was infused weekly as a 200 mg dose. The neuropathy symptom scores and the physicians global assessments improved compared with placebo ($P = 0.02$ and $P = 0.006$, respectively) [78].

Dr. Aaron Vinik has espoused the use of oral clonidine for small-fiber pain. He has recommended a bedtime dose of 0.1 mg and building slowly over several weeks to a dose of 0.5 mg. Most positive effects occur within the first 2 to 4 weeks. Patients need be cautioned about first-dose effect with orthostatic hypotension and dry mouth [79]. One other study proposes the use of transdermal clonidine in doses of 0.1 to 0.3 mg/week, but there have been no confirmatory trials [80].

Fifty-two patients were treated with sodium valproate for one month and there was a significant decrease in the McGill pain questionnaire (SF-MPQ) ($P < 0.05$) [81]. A recent trial in 41 patients who have hypertension, treated with the angiotensin-converting enzyme inhibitor (ACE) trandolapril, showed no change in neuropathic symptoms but improved peroneal motor nerve conduction velocity ($P = 0.03$), m-wave amplitude ($P = 0.03$), F-wave latency ($P = 0.03$), and the sural nerve action potential amplitude after 12 months [82]. Given ACE drugs effects on vascular endothelium and insulin resistance, one would expect them to improve nerve function, although ACE drugs will also increase bradykinin levels, which could potentially exacerbate underlying neuropathic symptoms [83]. Isosorbide dinitrate was used in an attempt to increase the availability of NO to the nerve and improve function. Twenty-two patients entered a double-blind, randomized, placebo-controlled trial with this medication. Neuropathic pain was reduced ($P < 0.02$), as was burning sensations ($P < 0.006$) [84]. Pentoxifylline showed no efficacy in a 6-month trial in 40 patients who have type 2 diabetes [85]. Kumar and Marshall described decreased pain in 15 of 18 patients treated for 30 minutes daily for 4 weeks with electrostimulation (H-wave machine, biphasic, exponentially decaying wave form, pulse width 4 ms, 25–35 V). In a follow-up report, these authors combined this transcutaneous stimulation with amitriptyline in patients in whom the drug had caused no or only partial pain relief. Again the treatment group showed improved pain relief [86,87].

Summary

Diabetes mellitus is a major health concern that is only expected to become more prevalent over the next few decades. It causes much morbidity and mortality through various macro- and microvascular complications, including diabetic neuropathy. Currently, there is no treatment that directly affects the natural course of diabetic neuropathy except for rigorous glycemic control, a goal that is not always achievable. Despite these therapeutic limitations, the morbidity caused by diabetic neuropathy can be minimized by early and accurate diagnosis. A detailed history and physical examination, along with carefully selected laboratory tests will confirm the presence of diabetic neuropathy while excluding other etiologies that may require alternative management strategies. Treatment is always tailored to the patient's symptoms. In addition to improved glycemic control, health care providers can provide education, support, and symptomatic relief. There are many pain modulating therapies that are effective in diabetic neuropathy as discussed above. Nortriptyline at low doses is an inexpensive well-tolerated medication that is effective. Gabapentin is an excellent choice when nortriptyline is ineffective or not tolerated. Other anticonvulsants, such as lamotrigine, carbamazepine, oxycarbazepine, and topiramate, may also provide benefit. Judicious use of narcotics is appropriate when other treatment modalities fail. The importance of treating underlying depression cannot be overemphasized. When gait becomes impaired as a result of neuropathy, appropriate prescription of assistive devices will prevent injuries from falls. Ankle-foot orthoses and other orthotic devices may allow patients to remain ambulatory and independent for a longer period. Despite the challenges ahead, the future holds the promise of more effective treatments for diabetes mellitus and its complications.

References

[1] The Hellmut Mehnert Award Workshop Participants. On your feet! Workshop on the diabetic foot. J Diabetes Complications 2002;16:183–94.
[2] Centers for Disease Control and Prevention. National diabetes fact sheet: national estimates and general information on diabetes in the United States. Atlanta (GA): US Department of Health and Human Services, Centers for Disease Control and Prevention; 1999.
[3] Proceedings of a consensus development conference on standardized measures in diabetic neuropathy. Diabetes Care 1992;15:1080–107.
[4] Harris M, Eastman R, Cowie C. Symptoms of sensory neuropathy in adults with NIDDM in the US population. Diabetes Care 1993;16(11):1446–52.
[5] Maser RE, Steenkiste AR, Dorman JS, et al. Epidemiological correlates of diabetic neuropathy: report from Pittsburgh Epidemiology of Diabetes Complications Study. Diabetes 1989; 38(11):1456.
[6] Dyck PJ, Kratz KM, Karnes JL, et al. The prevalence by staged severity of various types of diabetic neuropathy, retinopathy, and nephropathy in a population-based cohort: the Rochester Diabetic Neuropathy Study. Neurology 1993;43:817–24.
[7] Dyck PJ, et al. Variables influencing neuropathic endpoints. The Rochester Diabetic Neuropathy Study of Healthy Subjects. Neurology 1995;45:1115–21.
[8] Young MJ, Boulton AJM, Macleod AF, et al. A multicentre study of the prevalence of diabetic neuropathy in the United Kingdom hospital clinic population. Diabetologia 1993;36:150–4.
[9] Walter DP, Gatling W, Mullee MA, et al. The prevalence of diabetic distal sensory neuropathy in an English community. Diabet Med 1992;9(4):349.
[10] Veglio M, Sivieri R. Prevalence of neuropathy in IDDM patients in Piemonte, Italy. Diabetes Care 1993;16(2):456.

[11] Knuiman MW, Welborn TA, McCann VJ, et al. Prevalence of diabetic complications in relation to risk factors. Diabetes 1986;35(12):1332.
[12] Melton JL, Dyck PJ. Epidemiology. In: Dyck PJ, Thomas PK, editors. Diabetic neuropathy. 2nd edition. Philadelphia: W.B. Saunders; 1999. p. 239–54.
[13] Pirat J. Diabetes mellitus and its degenerative complications: a prospective study of 4,400 patients observed between 1947 and 1973. Part 1. Diabetes Care 1978;1(3):168.
[14] Pirat J. Diabetes mellitus and its degenerative complications: a prospective study of 4,400 patients observed between 1947 and 1973. Part 2. Diabetes Care 1978;1(4):252.
[15] The DCCT Research Group. The effect of intensive treatment of diabetes on the development and progression of long-term complications in insulin-dependent diabetes mellitus. N Engl J Med 1993;329:977–86.
[16] Dyck PJ, Lais A, Larnes JL, et al. Fiber loss is primary and multifocal in sural nerves in diabetic polyneuropathy. Ann Neurol 1986;19:425.
[17] Dyck PJB, Dyck PJ. Diabetic polyneuroapthy. In: Dyck PJ, Thomas PK, editors. Diabetic neuropathy. 2nd edition. Philadelphia: W.B. Saunders; 1999. p. 255–78.
[18] Taylor BV, Dyck PJ. Classification of the diabetic neuroapthies. In: Dyck PJ, Thomas PK, editors. Diabetic neuropathy. 2nd edition. Philadelphia: W.B. Saunders; 1999. p. 407–14.
[19] Smith BE. Cranial neuropathy in diabetes mellitus. In: Dyck PJ, Thomas PK, editors. Diabetic neuropathy. 2nd edition. Philadelphia: W.B. Saunders; 1999. p. 458.
[20] Boulton AJ, Drury J, Clarke D, Ward JD. Continuous subcutaneous insulin infusion in management of painful diabetic neuropathy. Diabetes Care 1982;5:386–90.
[21] Feldman EL, Stevens MJ, Thomas PK, et al. A practical two-step quantitative clinical and electrophysiological assessment for the diagnosis and staging of diabetic neuropathy. Diabetes Care 1994;17(11):1281–9.
[22] Tesfaye S, Malik R, Harris N, et al. Arterio-venous shunting and proliferating new vessels in acute painful neuropathy or rapid glycaemic control (insulin neuritis). Diabetalogia 1996;39:329–35.
[23] Simmons Z, Feldman EL. Update on diabetic neuropathy. Curr Opin Neurol 2002;15: 595–603.
[24] Dyck PJ, Hansen S, Karnes J, et al. Capillary number and percentage closed in human diabetic sural nerve. Proc Natl Acad Sci USA 1985;82:2513.
[25] Dyck PJ. Detection, characterization, and staging of polyneuropathy: assessed in diabetics. Muscle Nerve 1988;11:21–32.
[26] Edwards K, Glantz MJ, Button J. Efficacy and safety of topiramate in the treatment of painful diabetic neuropathy; a double-blind placebo-controlled trial [abstract]. Neurology 2000;S4:A81.
[27] Giannini A, Dyck PJ. Pathologic alterations in human diabetic neuroapthy. In: Dyck PJ, Thomas PK, editors. Diabetic neuropathy. 2nd edition. Philadelphia: W.B. Saunders; 1999. p. 279–96.
[28] Dyck PJ, Zimmerman IR, O'Brian PC, et al. Introduction of automated systems to evaluate touch-pressure, vibration, and thermal cutaneous sensation in man. Ann Neurol 1978;4:502.
[29] McQuay H, Carroll D, Jadad AR, et al. Anticonvulsant drugs for management of pain: a systematic review. BMJ 1995;311(7012):1047–52.
[30] Lozeron P, Nahu L, Lacroix C, et al. Symptomatic diabetic and non-diabetic neuropathies in a series of 100 diabetic patients. J Neurol 2002;249:569–75.
[31] Timperley WR, Boulton AJM, Davies-Jones GAB, et al. Small vessel disease in progressive diabetic neuropathy associated with good metabolic control. J Clin Pathol 1985;38:1030.
[32] Timperley WR, Ward JD, Preston FE, et al. Clinical and histological studies in diabetic neuropathy: a reassessment of vascular factors in relation to intravascular coagulation. Diabetologia 1976; 12:237.
[33] Vital C, LeBlanc M, Vallat JM, et al. Ultrastructural study of peripheral nerve in 16 diabetics without neuropathy: comparisons with 16 diabetic neuropathies and 16 non-diabetic neuropathies. Acta Neuropathologie (Berl) 1974;30:63.
[34] Willliams E, Timperley WR, Ward JD, et al. Electron microscopic studies of vessels in diabetic peripheral neuropathy. J Clin Pathol 1980;33:462.
[35] Brownlee M. Glycation and diabetic complications. Diabetes 1994;43(6):836–41.

[36] Johnson PC, Doll SC, Cromey DW. Pathogenesis of diabetic neuropathy. Ann Neurol 1986; 19:450.
[37] Feldman EL. Oxidative stress and diabetic neuropathy: a new understanding of an old problem. J Clin Invest 2003;111(4):431–3.
[38] Tanenberg RJ, Schumer MP, Greene D, Pfeifer MA. Neuropathic problems of lower extremities in diabetic patients. In: Bowker JH, Pfeifer MA, editors. Levin and O'Neal's: the diabetic foot. 6th edition. Philadelphia: Mosby; 2001. p. 33–64.
[39] Hata Y, Rook SL, Aiello LP. Basic fibroblast growth factor induces expression of VEGF receptor KDR through a protein kinase C and p44/p42 mitogen activated protein kinase-dependent pathway. Diabetes 1999;48:1145–55.
[40] Danis RP, Bingaman DP, Jirousek M, Yang Y. Inhibition of intraocular neovascularization caused by retinal ischemia in pigs by PKC-beta inhibition with LY33351. Invest Ophthalmol Vis Sci 1998; 39:171–9.
[41] The γ-Linolenic Acid Multicenter Trial Group. Treatment of diabetic neuropathy with γ-linolenic acid. Diabetes Care 1993;16:8–15.
[42] The DCCT Research Group. Ann Intern Med 1995;122(8):561–8.
[43] UKPDS 33. Intensive blood glucose control with sulfonylureas or insulin compared with conventional treatment and risk of complications in patients with type 2 diabetes mellitus. Lancet 1998; 352:837–53.
[44] Archer AG, Roberts VC, Thomas PK, et al. J Neurol Neurosurg Psychiatry 1983;46:491–9.
[45] Ziegler D, Mayer P, Muhlen H, Gries FA. Assessment of small and large fibre function-term type 1 (insulin-dependent) diabetic patients with and without diabetic neuropathy. Pain 1988;34: 1–10.
[46] Dejgard A, Petersen P, Kastrup J. Mexiletine for treatment of chronic painful diabetic neuropathy. Lancet 1988;1(8575–76):9–11.
[47] Apfel SC, Schwartz S, Adornato BT, et al. Efficacy and safety of recombinant nerve growth factor in patients with diabetic polyneuropathy: a randomized controlled trial. JAMA 2000;284(17): 2215–21.
[48] Stevens MJ, Feldman ML, Greene DA. The aetiology of diabetic neuropathy: the combined role of metabolic and vascular defects. Diabet Med 1995;12(7):566–79.
[49] Nicolucci A, Carcini F, Cavaliere D, et al. A meta-analysis of trials on aldose reductase inhibitors in diabetic peripheral neuropathy. Diabet Med 1996;13(12):1017–26.
[50] Ziegler D, Hanefield M, Ruthnau KJ, et al. Treatment of symptomatic peripheral sensory neuropathy with the anti-oxidant alpha lipoic acid. Diabetalogia 1995;38:1425–33.
[51] Melzack R, Wall PD. Pain mechanisms: a new theory. Science 1965;150:971–9.
[52] Ziegler D, Hanefield M, Ruthnau KJ, et al. Treatment of symptomatic polyneuropathy with the antioxidant alpha lipoic acid: a even month randomized controlled trial (ALADIN III study). Diabetes Care 1999;22:1296–301.
[53] Cohen KL, Harris S. Efficacy and safety of non-steroidal anti-inflammatory drugs in the therapy of diabetic neuropathy. Arch Intern Med 1987;147:1442–4.
[54] Harati Y, Gooch C, Swenson M, et al. Double-blind randomised trial of tramadol for the treatment of the pain of diabetic neuropathy. Neurology 1998;50(6):1842–6.
[55] Harati Y, et al. Maintenance of the long-term effectiveness of tramadol in the treatment of the pain of diabetic neuropathy. J Diabetes Comp 2000;14:65–70.
[56] Kvinesdal B, Molin J, Froland A, Gram LF. Imipramine treatment of painful diabetic neuropathy. JAMA 1984;251(13):1227–730.
[57] Max MB, Lynch SA, Muir J, et al. N Engl J Med 1992;326(19):1250–6.
[58] Davis JL, Lewis SB, Gerich JE, et al. JAMA 1977;238(21):2291–2.
[59] Sindrup SH, Gram LF, Brosen K, et al. Pain 1990;42(2):135–44.
[60] Davis JL, Smith RL. Painful peripheral diabetic neuropathy treated with venlafaxine HCL extended release capsules [letter]. Diabetes Care 1999;22:1909–10.
[61] Kiayias JA, Vlachou ED, Lakka-Papadodima E. Venlafaxine HCL in the treatment of painful peripheral diabetic neuropathy [letter]. Diabetes Care 2000;23:699.

[62] Lithner. Venlafaxine in treatment of severe painful peripheral diabetic neuropathy. Diabetes Care 2000;23:1710–1.
[63] Chadda VS, Mathur VS. Double-blind study of the effects of diphenylhydantoin sodium on diabetic neuropathy. J Assoc Phys India 1978;26:403–6.
[64] Saudek CD, Werns S, Reidenberg MM. Phenytoin in the treatment of symmetrical polyneuropathy. Clin Pharacol Ther 1977;22:196–9.
[65] Rull J, Quibrera R, Gonzalez-Millan H, Lozano Castanada O. Symptomatic treatment of peripheral diabetic neuropathy with carbamazepine (Tegretol): double-blind crossover study. Diabetalogia 1969;5:215–20.
[66] Chakrabarti AK, Samantaray SK. Diabetic peripheral neuropathy: nerve conduction studies before, during and after carbamazepine therapy. Aust N Z Med 1976;6(6):565–8.
[67] Tremont-Lukats IW, Megef C, Beckonja MM. Anti-convulsants for neuropathic pain syndromes—mechanism of action and place ion therapy. Drugs 2000;60:1029–52.
[68] Backonja M, Beydoun A, Edwards KR, et al. Gabapentin for the symptomatic treatment of painful neuropathy in patients with diabetes mellitus: a randomized-controlled trial. JAMA 1998;280(21): 1831–6.
[69] Morel CM, Neckband SG, Stoner CP, et al. Randomized double-blind study comparing the efficacy of gabapentin with amitriptyline on diabetic peripheral neuropathy pain. Arch Intern Med 1999; 159(16):1931–7.
[70] Eisenberg E, Alon N, Ishay A, et al. Lamotrigine in the treatment of painful diabetic neuropathy. Eur J Neurol 1998;5:167–73.
[71] Eisenberg E, Lurie Y, Braker C, et al. Lamotrigine reduces painful diabetic neuropathy. Neurology 2001;57:505–9.
[72] Kastrup J, Petersen P, Dejard A, et al. Intravenous lidocaine infusion: a new treatment of chronic painful diabetic neuropathy. Pain 1987;28:69–75.
[73] Oskarsson P, Ljungren JG, Lins PE. Efficacy and safety of mexiletine in the treatment of painful diabetic neuropathy. The mexiletine study group. Diabetes Care 1997;20(10): 1594–7.
[74] Stracke H, Meyer UE, Schumacher HE, Federlin K. Mexiletine in the treatment of diabetic neuropathy. Diab Care 1992;15(11):1550–5.
[75] Wright JM, Oki JC, Graves L. Mexiletine in the symptomatic treatment of diabetic peripheral neuropathy. Ann Pharmacol Ther 1997;31:29–34.
[76] Capsaicin Study Group. Effect of treatment with capsaicin on daily activities of patients with painful diabetic neuropathy. Diabetes Care 1992;15(2):159–65.
[77] Zhang WY, Wan Po AL. The effectiveness of topically applied capsaicin: a meta-analysis. Eur J Clin Pharm 1994;46:517–22.
[78] Amin P, Sturrock NDC. A pilot study of the beneficial effects of amantadine in the treatment of painful diabetic peripheral neuropathy. Diab Med 2003;20(2):114–8.
[79] Vinik AI. Managing the pain of diabetic neuropathy. Medscape Diabetes Endocrinology 2001;3(1).
[80] Byas-Smith MG, Max MB, Muir J, Kingman A. Transdermal clonidine compared to placebo in painful diabetic neuropathy using a two-stage "enriched enrollment" design. Pain 1995;60: 267–74.
[81] Kochar DK, Jain N, Agarwal RP, et al. Sodium valproate in the management of painful neuropathy in type 2 diabetes—a randomized placebo controlled study. Acta Neurol Scand 2002; 106(5):248–52.
[82] Malik RA, Williamson S, Abbott C, et al. Effect of angiotensin converting enzyme inhibitor trandolapril on human diabetic neuropathy: randomised double blind controlled trial. Lancet 1998;352(9145):1978–81.
[83] Spruce MC, Potter J, Coppini DV. The pathogenesis and management of painful diabetic neuropathy review. Diabet Med 2003;20:88–98.
[84] Cohen SM, Matthews T. Pentoxifylline in the treatment of distal diabetic neuropathy. Angiology 1991;42(9):741–6.

[85] Yuen KCJ, Baker NR, Raman G. Treatment of chronic painful diabetic neuropathy with isosorbide dinitrate spray. Diab Care 2003;25:1699–703.
[86] Kumar D, Alvaro MS, Julka AS, Marshall HJ. Diabetic peripheral neuropathy: effectiveness of electrotherapy and amitriptyline for symptomatic relief. Diabetes Care 1998;21(8):1322–5.
[87] Kumar D, Marshall HJ. Diabetic peripheral neuropathy: amelioration of pain with transcutaneous electrostimulation. Diabetes Care 1997;20(11):1702–5.

CLINICS IN PODIATRIC MEDICINE AND SURGERY

Clin Podiatr Med Surg
20 (2003) 689–708

Vascular evaluation and arterial reconstruction of the diabetic foot

Bauer E. Sumpio, MD, PhD[a,*], Taeseung Lee, MD[a], Peter A. Blume, DPM[b]

[a]Yale University School of Medicine, Department of Surgery (Vascular), 333 Cedar Street, FMB 137, New Haven, CT 06510, USA

[b]Yale-New Haven Hospital, 20 York Street, New Haven, CT 06510, USA

Ulceration of diabetic feet pose a major threat to limb integrity and account for more than 20% of hospital admissions in patients who have diabetes and an estimated annual health care cost of more than $1 billion [1–3]. Failure of these ulcers to heal leads to lower extremity amputations. In addition, nearly half of all patients who undergo amputation will develop limb-threatening ischemia in the contralateral limb and many will ultimately require an amputation of the opposite limb within 5 years [4].

The pathophysiologic mechanisms underlying diabetic foot disease include neuropathy, infection, and ischemia [3,5]. Although peripheral neuropathy has a central role and is present in over 80% of diabetic foot lesions [6,7], inadequate perfusion will always result in a nonhealing wound [1,8]. Lower extremity ischemia due to vascular disease reduces the pedal supply of oxygen, nutrients, and soluble mediators that are involved in the repair process [9]. Lack of arterial blood flow decreases tissue resilience, leads to rapid death of tissue, and impedes wound healing. Correction of hypoxia improves cutaneous microcirculation in the neuropathic diabetic foot, resulting in retardation of the progression of neuropathy [10,11]. It is therefore necessary to perform a vascular assessment on all patients who have foot ulcers (Box 1).

This work was supported in part by the North American Foundation for Limb Preservation.

* Corresponding author.
E-mail address: bauer.sumpio@yale.edu (B.E. Sumpio).

doi:10.1016/S0891-8422(03)00088-0

Box 1. Evaluation of the diabetic foot

History taking
Physical examination
- Inspection
- Ulcer location
- Appearance
- Depth of penetration
- Pedal pulse palpation

Radiography to detect
- Osteomyelitis
- Subcutaneous gas

Vascular evaluation

General assessment

The assessment of patients with diabetes begins with a complete history and physical examination. Asymptomatic patients with multiple identified atherosclerotic risk factors should be routinely screened for involvement of the peripheral vasculature. Ten percent of individuals aged 55 to 74 years have asymptomatic lower extremity arterial disease when screened [12]. Furthermore, atherosclerotic occlusive disease is but one manifestation of a generalized process with affected individuals often presenting with concomitant lesions in a variety of vascular beds, such as the coronary, carotid, or renal vasculature [13–15].

The symptoms of arterial insufficiency occur as a result of inadequate perfusion to the lower extremity musculature relative to its metabolism with the affected ischemic tissue producing pain. Patients may complain of an acute onset of symptoms, have chronic complaints, or have acute symptoms superimposed on chronic complaints. The patient with identifiable atherosclerotic risk factors may complain of the sudden onset of extremity pain associated with coolness and variable numbness as a manifestation of acute thrombosis of an already involved segment or embolism from more proximal sources. On a more chronic basis, the patient may complain of pain in the buttocks or calves brought on with activity and relieved with rest (intermittent claudication), burning pain in the forefoot aggravated by elevation and relieved by dependency (rest pain), or the development of ulceration on the legs, feet, or between the toes. Multilevel atherosclerotic disease is usually required to produce significant symptomatology. The classical symptoms of claudication or rest pain may be obscured by neuropathy in the patient who has diabetes, and the visual identification of ulcers may be delayed because of associated visual loss from diabetic retinopathy. Elderly patients with significant cardiac or pulmonary disease may not be sufficiently ambulatory to trigger complaints of claudication even though significant disease may be present.

Other important historical information will influence decision making, including the patient's past medical, surgical, ambulatory, and nutritional histories. Ten percent of patients with lower extremity arterial disease have cerebrovascular disease and 28% have coronary heart disease, emphasizing the need to identify comorbidities. In addition, allergic reactions to medications should be documented with specific attention to iodinated contrast agents and shellfish, which may impact on the ability to safely perform contrast angiography.

Vascular examination

A complete vascular examination can only be performed with the patient supine in an examination gown. The patient's temperature, respiratory rate, heart rate, and blood pressure in both upper extremities are recorded and abnormalities noted. Fever may indicate the presence of an infected ulcer, and the presence of tachycardia and tachypnea may support the diagnosis of a septic foot. A 15 mmHg difference in arm pressures signifies occlusive disease in the subclavian-axillary segment.

The signs of arterial insufficiency will vary depending on the chronicity and severity of the problem. Visual inspection coupled with an accurate history will determine the presence of a chronic vascular condition. The color of the skin is conferred by blood in the subpapillary layer and will vary with the position of the extremity, temperature of the skin, and degree of blood oxygenation (reduced hemoglobin → blue). In chronic arterial insufficiency, the arterioles will maximally dilate as a compensatory response to the chronic ischemia intensifying color changes. During acute arterial occlusion, the venules will empty, leading to a chalky white appearance regardless of extremity position. Partial but inadequate perfusion from an incomplete acute or chronic occlusion allows for pooling of blood in the venules, which may be red in cold temperatures or blue at higher temperatures. When the extremity is at the level of the heart, the pooled blood masks the arterial flow. Elevation of the extremity above the level of the central venous pressure (rarely greater than 25 cm) allows the pooled venous blood to drain, allowing an accurate assessment of the degree of arterial flow. The normal extremity will remain pink, whereas that with arterial insufficiency will become pallid. Conversely, allowing the extremity to become dependent will cause an intense rubor or cyanosis (dependent rubor). The time of return of blood to the dependent extremity is a useful marker of the severity of the deficit (normally less than 20 seconds). With a diminished nutritional supply to the skin there is thinning and functional loss of the dermal appendages evident as dry, shiny, and hairless skin. The nails may become brittle and ridged. Comparison of color and trophic changes between extremities gives a good indication of the severity of the process unless a bilateral deficit is present, in which case the experience of the examiner will be required to make an accurate diagnosis.

Skin temperature is a reliable indicator of the blood flow rate in the dermal vessels, though flow is governed primarily by constriction or dilation of the arterioles to maintain a constant core temperature. Nevertheless, the temperature of the skin as a marker of perfusion is useful and can be assessed by lightly palpating the skin with the back of the hand and comparing similar sites from one extremity to the other. An ischemic limb is cool, and demarcation of temperature gives a rough indication of the level of the occlusion. Again, assessment of temperature differences is confounded when both extremities are affected.

Extremity ulcerations have a characteristic appearance depending on their etiology (Fig. 1) [1,16]. Ulcerations caused by ischemia are typically located at the most distal end of the arterial system and are most commonly found on the tips of the toes and between the digits (Fig. 1A). The lesions often appear punched out and are painful but exhibit little bleeding. Neuropathic ulcerations typically occur at the heel (Fig. 1B) or over the metatarsal heads on the plantar surface (mal perforans ulcer) (Fig. 1C) but may also occur in less characteristic locations secondary to trauma or pressure. The associated sensory neuropathy in the patient who has diabetes may allow the destructive process to go unchecked such that extension into the deep plantar space can occur with minimal symptomatology. It is important to differentiate the rubor associated with vascular insufficiency and cellulitis accompanying an infective process. Cellulitic color changes will persist despite extremity elevation. In addition to ulcers, patients may present with a

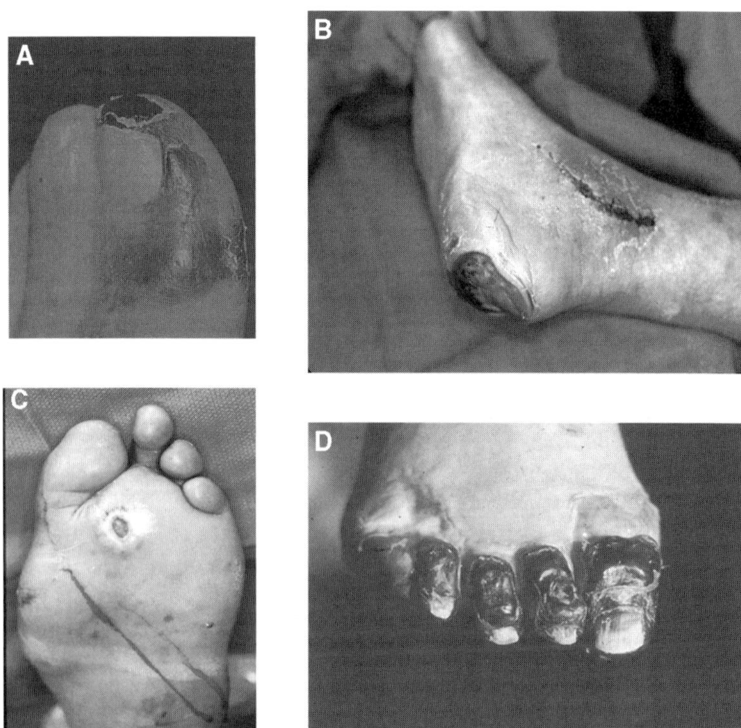

Fig. 1. Extremity ulcers. (*A*) Toe ulcer. (*B*) Calcaneal ulcer. (*C*) Plantar ulcer overlying metatarsal heads. (*D*) Forefoot gangrene.

varying degrees of tissue loss or frankly gangrenous digits, forefoot, or hindfoot. The presence of dry gangrene is a stable process allowing for a complete vascular evaluation; however, any progression to an infected wet gangrene requires immediate surgical debridement (Fig. 1D).

Noninvasive vascular lab

The noninvasive vascular laboratory plays an important role in the care of patients who have diabetes [12,17]. Current noninvasive vascular tests include physiologic and anatomic testing modalities (Box 2). Segmental limb pressures, Doppler and plethysmographic waveform analysis, transcutaneous oximetry, and skin perfusion pressure all provide important functional information on the adequacy of perfusion. Color duplex imaging provides more specific anatomic and physiologic information. In the presence of diabetes, however, many of the physiologic tests have significant limitations. A common finding in patients who have diabetes or long-standing renal insufficiency is the presence of medial calcinosis of peripheral arteries. The artery is less compressible, and indirect measurement of pressure within the vessel is artificially increased when compression is performed.

Limb pressure measurements

Segmental limb pressures are an extension of the bedside ankle-brachial index. This noninvasive test is indicated in any patient for whom history and physical examination suggests peripheral vascular disease. By obtaining pressures at successive levels of the extremity, the level of disease can be localized in most cases.

The patient is placed in a supine position and rested for 15 minutes, at which point four standard-sized blood pressure cuffs are placed at the high thigh, above-knee, below-knee, and ankle positions (Fig. 2). The dorsalis pedis or posterior tibial arterial Doppler signal is obtained with a continuous wave Doppler at the ankle, and the pressure at each cuff level that occludes the pedal signal is measured by first inflating the cuff until the signal is no longer heard and then progressively deflating the cuff until the signal resumes. The pressure at each level is divided by the highest systolic arm pressure to obtain an index for each level. The proximal thigh pressure is usually recorded to be 30 to 40 mmHg higher than the brachial pressure, though in reality in the normal individual these pressures should be nearly equal. This artifact occurs because the thigh cuff width is often not

Box 2. Noninvasive vascular laboratory

- Toe brachial pressure measurement
- Waveform analysis
- Color duplex imaging
- Transcutaneous oxygen measurement

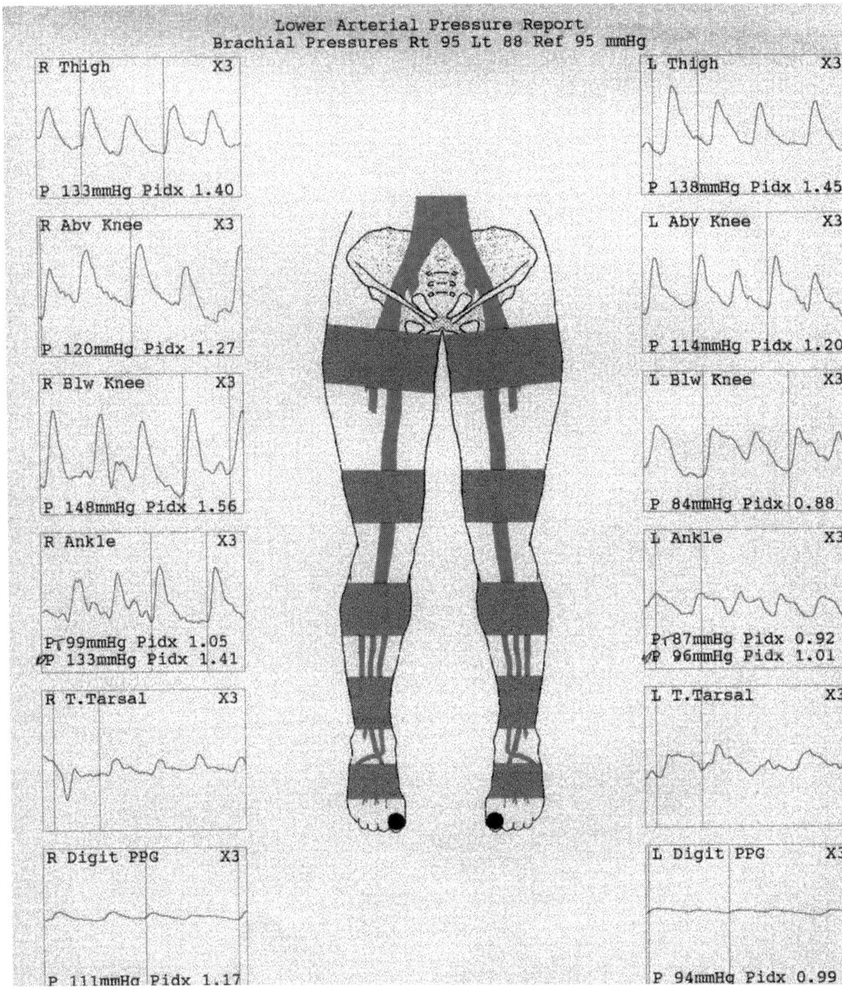

Fig. 2. Physiologic measurement of perfusion to lower extremity with pulse volume recordings and segmental pressures.

appropriately 120% the diameter of the limb at the thigh level to provide an accurate pressure reading. A high thigh index less than 1.2 is considered abnormal and may reflect aorto-iliac disease of concomitant profunda and superficial femoral obstruction, depending on the placement of the cuff relative to these structures. However, a normal high-thigh brachial index rules out aortoiliac disease. Differences in index level between the cuff levels as well as between each extremity at the same level are made. A 20-mmHg pressure gradient between successive levels on the same extremity is considered a significant pressure drop and correlates with flow-limiting vascular lesions. Successive significant decrements indicate multilevel disease. Comparison of the unaffected with the affected limb is a good indicator of the severity of the process; the systolic pressures measured at the same level in both legs normally should not differ by more than 20 mmHg. Pressure gradients may be increased in the hypertensive patient and decreased in low cardiac output states. Adequate collateralization may also diminish the observed pressure gradient, obscuring a significant lesion. Segmental pressure measurements are useful in the serial evaluation of patients over time and are reliable as an assessment of changes relative to risk factor intervention, exercise programs, or revascularization. Any change in index greater than 0.15 at the same cuff level from one study to the next is considered significant.

Toe pressures

Diabetics with medial sclerosis and patients with chronic renal insufficiency often have nonocclusive pressures with ABIs greater than 1.3, limiting the usefulness of segmental pressures in the evaluation of peripheral vascular disease in these populations. Toe digital arteries are less likely to be calcified, so that toe occlusive pressure measurements more reliably reflect pressure within the digital artery. Therefore, the toe brachial index (TBI) is a more reliable indicator of foot perfusion in diabetics [12].

A pneumatic cuff is placed on the digit and a photoelectrode placed on the end of the digit to obtain a photoplethysmographic (PPG) arterial waveform. An infrared light is transmitted into the superficial layers of the skin and the reflected portion is received by a phototransistor within the plethysmographic sensor. The resulting signal is proportional to the quantity of red blood cells in the cutaneous circulation Analogous to the segmental cuff pressures, the toe cuff is inflated until the waveform flattens and is then progressively deflated. The systolic pressure is recorded at the point in which the normal waveform is reestablished. The ratio of the recorded systolic pressure to the higher of the two brachial pressures gives the toe-brachial index (Fig. 2). The absolute toe pressures are of value in the estimation of the healing potential ulcer, with a pressure greater than 30 mm Hg favorable for ulcer healing [18–21]. Though toe pressures are useful to define perfusion at the level of the foot in those with incompressible vessels, no indication of the level of disease is obtained.

Pulse volume recordings (PVR)

An adjunctive method to establish the disease level in these individuals is through waveform analysis with pulse volume recordings (PVR) or Doppler waveform. PVR is the most commonly used waveform analysis and is less operator dependent than Doppler waveform analysis [22].

Pulse volume recordings are obtained through the application of sequential blood pressure cuffs with an air pleythysmographic technique. Each cuff is inflated (10–65 mmHg) and variations in blood volume in the tissue beneath the cuff can be indirectly assessed through the alterations in pressure transmitted through the inflated cuff to a pressure transducer that records the variations through the cardiac cycle to produce a waveform (Fig. 2). Conversion of this pressure signal to an appropriately calibrated electrical signal permits production of an analog tracing that can be examined and interpreted. The normal PVR waveform has a sharp upstroke and peak with a reflected wave present before returning to baseline. With mild obstruction, the reflected wave is lost, the upstroke delayed, and the peak blunted. Moderate to severe obstruction produces a bowing of the downstroke away from the baseline. A flat PVR is irregular with low amplitude and indicates severe obstruction.

Exercise testing

Segmental blood pressure testing, toe brachial index measurements, and waveform analysis can be performed before and after exercise to unmask occlusive disease not apparent on resting studies. With exercise, blood flow normally increases three to fivefold to meet the increased demand and resistance in the muscular bed falls. The presence of a significant stenosis limits this compensatory response and magnifies the pressure gradient across the lesion. The standard test involves walking on the treadmill at 2 miles per hour at 12% grade for 5 minutes or until the patient is forced to stop. The walking time and nature of symptoms are recorded. The magnitude of the decrease in ankle systolic pressure and time for recovery to resting pressure are evaluated. The ABI is recorded at rest, 1 minute after exercise, and every minute thereafter until the baseline level is returned; the pressure in patients with severe disease may not return to baseline within the allotted time for the test. A normal response to exercise is a slight increase or no change in the ankle systolic pressure compared with baseline and rules out vascular insufficiency as the cause of symptoms. A fall in ankle pressure by more than 20% of baseline or below an absolute pressure of 60 mmHg that requires more than 3 minutes to recover is considered abnormal. Single-level disease is inferred with a recovery time less than 6 minutes; greater than a 6-minute recovery time is associated with multilevel disease.

The administration of pharmacologic agents, such as priscoline, or the induction of reactive hyperemia can be performed in place of exercise testing in patients with limited exercise ability due to cardiopulmonary disease of musculoskeletal problems. Reactive hyperemia testing involves the placement of a pneumatic cuff at the thigh level to suprsaystolic pressure for 3 to 5 minutes, producing ischemia and compensatory vasodilation distal to the cuff. The changes that occur upon release of the cuff are similar to those obtained with treadmill testing. Normally a transient 25% drop in ankle pressure does occur, unlike treadmill testing. Single-level arterial disease is indicated by a drop in ankle pressure less than 50%, whereas a greater than 50% drop is seen in multilevel disease.

Transcutaneous oximetry

Transcutaneous oxygen (TcPO2) tension may provide supplemental information regarding local tissue perfusion and is often used to assess the healing potential

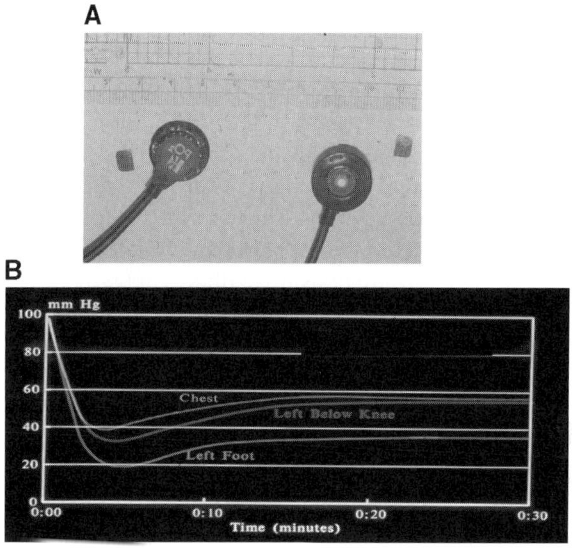

Fig. 3. Transcutaneous oximetry. (*A*) Platinum oxygen electrodes. (*B*) TcPO2 tracing.

of lower extremity ulcers or amputation sites [23]. Previous studies showed that TcPO2 measurements can accurately predict severity of foot ischemia and can be used to select appropriate treatment (conservative versus operative) for patients with diabetes [24]. Platinum oxygen electrodes are placed on the chest wall and legs or feet (Fig. 3). Either the absolute value at the oxygen tension at the foot or leg or a ratio of this value to that of the chest wall may be evaluated. A normal value at the foot is 60 mmHg and a normal chest/foot ratio is 0.9. Controversy exists regarding the optimal level for tissue healing. It is generally accepted that wounds are likely to heal if oxygen tension is greater than 40 mmHg (foot/chest ratio greater than 0.5) and that healing is not likely to with a value less than 20 mmHg [25].

Transcutaneous oxygen measurements can also be obtained in conjunction with exercise testing. Normally the value will not diminish; however, in the patient with arterial occlusive disease, the value will fall. A higher value must be achieved for healing of an ulcer in the diabetic foot. The accuracy of the value obtained is limited by local edema, skin temperature, emotional state (sympathetic vasoconstriction), and pharmacologic agents.

Duplex imaging

The routine evaluation of waveforms in conjunction with segmental pressures and segmental indices increase the accuracy of Doppler testing. Color duplex imaging incorporates real-time B-mode imaging, and pulsed and color Doppler. Real time B-mode imaging allows for vessel identification and anatomic detail of the vessel. Color Doppler imaging provides for the direction of flow and the presence of turbulence. In addition, degree of diameter reduction or stenosis is calculated by peak systolic velocity and velocity ratios.

Real-time ultrasonography uses reflected sound waves to produce images and assess blood velocity. Two ultrasound modes are routinely used in vascular imaging, the B (brightness) mode and the Doppler mode (B mode imaging + Doppler flow detection = duplex ultrasound). Both of these modes take advantage of pulsed sound waves to distinguish them from the continuous wave hand-held ultrasound probe, which requires two ultrasound crystals, one for sending and one for receiving sound waves. Continuous wave ultrasound provides a signal that is a summation of all the vascular structures through which the sound has passed and hence is limited in the evaluation of a specific vascular structure when multiple vessels are present. The amplitude of the audible signal can be interpreted, and the triphasic, biphasic, and monophasic nature of these signals appreciated. Pulsed wave technology uses a row of crystals, each of which alternately send and receive pulse trains of sound waves with a slight time delay with respect to their adjacent crystals. The time and intensity differences of the transmitted and received sound waves are converted to an image that displays depth and intensity for each crystal in the row (B mode). The identification of vascular structures from the B-mode display is enhanced in the color mode that displays movement (blood flow) within the field. Flow toward the transducer is red and flow away from the transducer is blue; the colors are semiquantitative and do not represent actual arterial and venous flow. The frequency shift between the transmitted and received sound waves caused by movement within the field is analyzed to generate velocity information (Doppler mode). Accurate velocity measurements require proper positioning of the ultrasound probe relative to the direction of flow at 60 degrees, ideally; however, between 30 and 70 degrees is acceptable. The velocity of blood within the vessel can be obtained and a calculation of the ratio of the velocity at a suspected stenosis to a normal portion of the vessel calculated. The ultrasound machine also performs a complex mathematical manipulation (Fourier transformation) to convert the sound information into frequency information. The characteristics of the resulting spectral waveform also provide useful information that can be used to estimate the severity of disease within the vessel. Arterial and venous disease can be assessed using duplex scanning.

The normal arterial waveform is triphasic with a sharp upstroke, a sharp peak during systole, a sharp downstroke, a reversed flow component, and forward diastolic flow. Progressive obstructive lesions cause a loss of reversed flow or of the forward diastolic flow, resulting in a biphasic signal. Decreased peripheral vascular resistance is responsible for the loss of the diastolic flow component and may be normal in older patients or reflect compensatory vasodilation in response to obstructive vascular lesions. The monophasic signal is characterized by a delayed upstroke, blunted peak, and no second component. Severe obstruction leads to a flat waveform. Progressive spectral broadening is also seen with increasing lesion severity.

The role of duplex ultrasound scanning as a screening test in vascular patients is well established. With increasing frequency, patients who require vascular procedure, such as carotid endarterectomy, are being safely treated based on duplex findings alone. However, in terms of duplex arterial mapping in lower extremities, there remains considerable debate regarding its accuracy [26,27]. Color duplex imaging appears effective for assessment of occlusive disease of the lower extremities, especially above knee, but may be less reliable in the infrapopliteal segments. Duplex scanning is useful in the evaluation of the vasculature pre- and postoperatively for graft surveillance. Up to 30% of bypass grafts will develop hyperplastic lesions, which, when appropriately detected and repaired by duplex scanning, results in improved long-term patency.

Vascular imaging

Intravenous contrast angiography continues to be the gold standard for imaging of the blood vessels and has been reserved traditionally for anatomic assessment before a planned intervention (Fig. 4). Because atheromatous plaques are often asymmetric and eccentric, multiple planar views must be obtained to estimate the severity of a stenotic lesion. Recognizable patterns of atherosclerotic occlusive disease occur with luminal lesions commonly present at the ostia of branch vessels or at bifurcations. The presence of atherogenic risk factors over a period of time results in involvement of multiple levels of disease. As a rule, younger patients tend to have isolated aortoiliac and focal SFA disease, whereas older patients present with a more diffuse distribution of atherosclerotic disease with involvement of the popliteal and tibial vessels. Diabetes mellitus predisposes the patient to isolated tibial/peroneal lesions and a tendency toward more diffuse profunda femoral disease, less aortoiliac involvement, and often sparing the SFA and popliteal arteries. Therefore, severe tibial occlusive disease can preclude visualization of distal runoff vessels. Technical modification, including selective catheter injection or direct intraarterial injection of a vasodilato,r might be helpful to visualize pedal vessels.

Previous studies have shown that graft patency correlates with visualization of pedal arch [28,29]. Inadequate visualization of the crural artery by angiography may lead to unnecessary amputation. If the Doppler examination suggests patent vessels in the distal leg, the use of preoperative or intraoperative antegrade arteriography may enhance distant vessel visualization that could lead to limb salvage. With current arteriographic techniques, more than 90% of patients who have diabetes presenting with ischemic foot lesions are shown to have surgically correctable occlusive disease [30]. The formation of collateral vessels is apparent in those with chronic disease, and the absence of collateral vessels associated with abrupt contrast cut-offs or filling defects suggest arterial embolization. Aneurysms might be inferred from an enlarged lumen; however, when partially thrombosed they may be difficult to visualize. Additional imaging with duplex ultrasonography is suggested. Arterial wall medial calcification can be demonstrated on scout films, before the injection with IV contrast, and the severity estimated.

Recently, the classic concept of contrast angiography before surgery has been challenged with the suggestion that some interventions can be undertaken

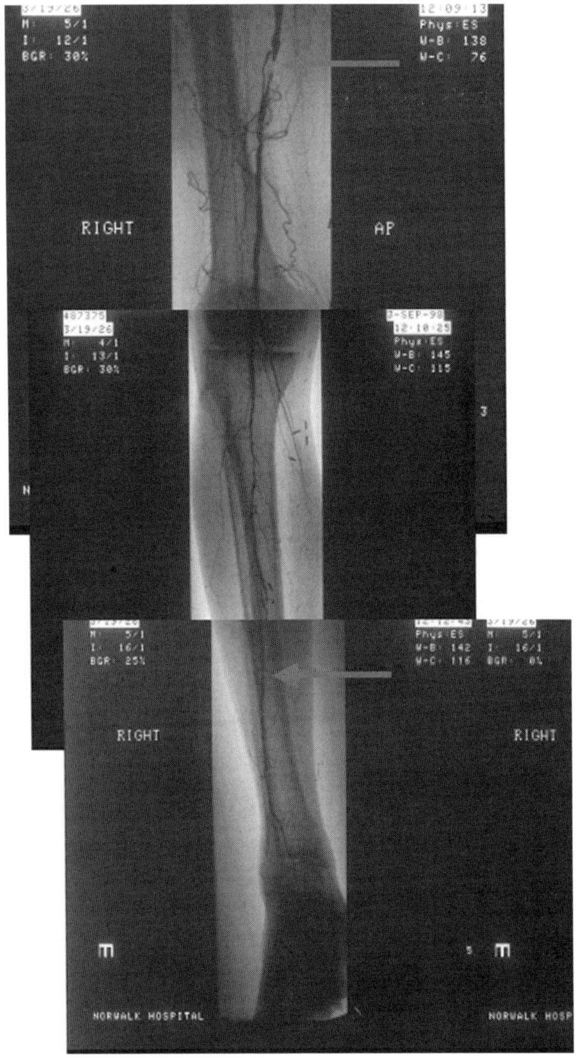

Fig. 4. Lower extremity angiogram. Arrows identify areas of stenosis.

with information gained from duplex scanning alone. The advantage of contrast angiography over noninvasive methods of vascular assessment is in the potential for intervention at the time of the study.

Another concern for patients who have diabetes is the possibility of the development of renal failure induced by the contrast agent [31,32]. The incidence of renal failure can be minimized by hydration before angiography [33,34]. Before the angiography, the patient is gently hydrated to minimize renal complications with attention to their medical history and ability to tolerate a fluid load. A carefully performed vascular exam is documented and baseline laboratory values obtained

(BUN, creatinine, PT/PTT, hemoglobin, and platelet). Abnormal coagulation parameters are corrected and any allergic reactions to IV contrast are ascertained. Intraarterial digital subtraction angiography is able to produce excellent angiograms, even in the distal pedal circulation, with a minimal amount of contrast.

Magnetic resonance imaging

Magnetic resonance angiography (MRA) is another imaging modality that can be used instead of contrast angiography (Fig. 5) [35,36]. The identification of patent runoff vessels in crural foot regions is necessary to perform successful bypass in patients who have diabetes. An advantage of MRA over conventional angiography is that the visualization of vessels depends on blood flow alone, not on the delivery of intravascular contrast media. The arrival of an aortic injection of contrast media distal to severe stenosis, mostly observed in patients who have diabetes, can be markedly delayed and diluted by the collateral supply; the slow flow within these vessels is readily detected by MRA. Several studies have shown that MRA has greater sensitivity than conventional angiography in the identification of distal runoff vessels [37,38]. MRA also serves as a supplemental method to assess the vasculature in patients with severe IV contrast allergy, contrast-induced nephropathy, or severe inflow disease and slow distal flow. MRA can display reconstructed images as conventional arteriograms with excellent demonstration of the infrainguinal arteries, including the small vessels of the foot. It is particularly useful for visualization of the distal vessels of the leg and foot in patients with severe proximal occlusive disease. One of the limitations of conventional angiog-

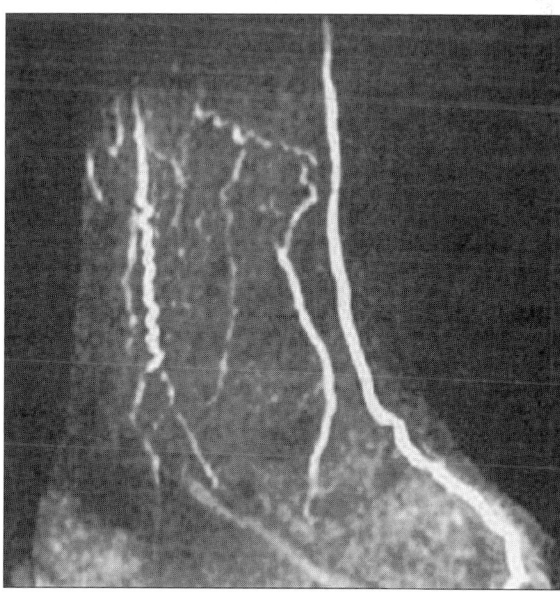

Fig. 5. Magnetic resonance angiogram of the foot.

raphy has been the failure to opacify the distal vasculature in those patients with severe inflow disease despite enhancement with the use of vasodilators, delayed filming, reactive hyperemia, or digital subtraction arteriography. This restriction is inherent to the technique whereby proximally injected contrast medium must traverse multiple segmental occlusions before opacifying the distal bed. MRA has been shown to be more sensitive in identifying patent vessels at all levels in patients with severe disease with the greatest difference seen in the distal vasculature. MRA can also be used to quantitate the degree of arterial stenosis with a reasonable degree of correlation to conventional angiography and has also been used to measure blood flow velocities. With continued improvements in computer based imaging, enhanced speed, resolution, and decreased cost, MR-based technology may one day usurp conventional angiography from its current diagnostic role and relegate it to primarily interventional procedures.

Arterial reconstruction

Lower extremity ischemia is classified according to the location of the arterial obstruction relative to the inguinal ligament. Ischemic symptoms can result from aortoiliac occlusive lesions (inflow disease) or femoropopliteal occlusive lesions (outflow disease). Despite extensive medial calcification of the aortoiliac system, patients who have diabetes do not usually have significant isolated aortoiliac occlusive disease. Ischemic rest pain in patients with such proximal disease is uncommon because of the extensive collateral network that develops. However, patients with aortoiliac occlusive disease will commonly demonstrate concomitant obstructive arteriopathy in the femoropoliteal or infrapopliteal segment. Generally, correction of hemodynamically significant inflow lesions will result in substantive improvement in symptoms in all genders [39–42].

A thorough understanding of the patterns of lower extremity ischemia in patients who have diabetes is fundamental to the rational application of distal surgical revascularization. The patient may present with gangrene of the toe secondary to the ischemia of the digital arteries or pressure gangrene and still have adequate flow to the level of the dorsalis pedis artery or posterior tibial artery. Most reported series of femoropopliteal reconstruction show an incidence of diabetes of around 40%. Although most patients who have rest pain or gangrene will have infrapopliteal occlusive arterial disease, some patients might have isolated femoropopliteal occlusive disease. In patients with simple occlusion of the superficial femoral artery, surgical bypass or percutaneous transluminal angioplasty (PTA) can be selected. Although many surgeons prefer the use of autogenous vein for bypass, polytetrafluroethylene (PTFE) grafts have been used liberally for above-knee femoropopliteal bypasses. The rationale for this option is to save the saphenous vein for the possible need for a later distal reconstruction, especially in patients who have diabetes, who commonly develop progressive popliteal disease. Advancement in the understanding of the etiology of graft failure has also led to improvements in the design and construct of these prosthetic vascular conduits [43].

The incidence of infrapopliteal vascular occlusive disease in the patient who has diabetes is higher than in the nondiabetic population [44]. However, patients who have diabetes tend to have less occlusive arterial disease in the foot than nondiabetics [44,45]. Given the unique pattern of peripheral atherosclerosis in patients who have diabetes, it is important during arteriography to study the foot vessels even when the three infragenicular arteries are occluded. A common error is to abort arteriography when occlusion of the three crural arteries is seen, presuming that all downstream vessels are also occluded.

Lower extremity occlusive arterial diseases frequently requires a bypass from an inflow vessel, usually the femoral artery, to a reconstituting outflow target (eg, the tibial or peroneal artery). Often, in diabetics, bypass grafting to the popliteal or tibioperoneal arteries cannot accomplish this goal because of more distal arterial disease. Similarly, although excellent results have been reported with peroneal bypass grafting [46], the peroneal artery is not in direct continuity with the foot vessels, and thus maximal flow to the foot may not be achieved. A fundamental principal in treating diabetics with foot ulcers is to provide maximal perfusion to the foot. Frequently, this can be achieved with vein graft bypass to the dorsalis pedis artery, posterior tibialis, and even the more distal tarsal arteries (Fig. 6). Autogenous vein grafting to these pedal vessels represents a technical advance that provides durable and effective limb salvage [47,48]. Bypass grafts to the dorsalis pedis artery, for example, can provide substantial perfusion to the ischemic heel lesion comparable with forefoot lesions [30]. Although it is possible to bypass to the posterior tibial artery, its use is sometimes limited in patients who have diabetes by significant tibial atherosclerosis. In addition, if there are no lesions in the superficial femoral or popliteal artery, a short-vein bypass can be accomplished

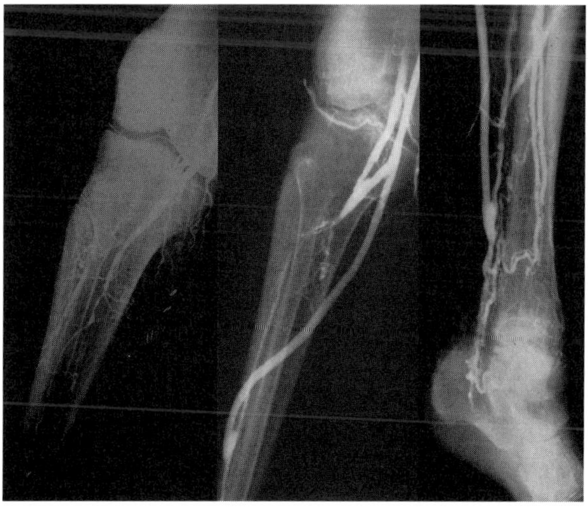

Fig. 6. Completion arteriogram of distal bypass to the foot. Panel 1: Bypass to politeal artery below the knee. Panel 2: Bypass to popliteal artery and anterior tibial artery. Panel 3: Distal bypass to posterior tibial artery.

from one of those arteries as a inflow with long-term patency [49,50]. A bypass originating from the popliteal artery is a frequent therapeutic option because of the short nature of the bypass [51].

Key to the success of pedal bypass procedures is the availability and quality of an autogenous vein for use as a conduit. Sometimes only a short segment of suitable autogenous vein may be available because patients have undergone coronary artery bypass grafting or previous lower extremity bypass. Innovative uses of prosthetic or composite grafts are required to aggressively salvage diabetic limbs. Fundamental elements of successful bypass are meticulous technique, including careful dissection, preservation of arterial tributaries, and use of magnifying loops to ensure properly constructed anastamosis that have a durable patency.

Role of endovascular therapy

The incorporation of endovascular techniques into the vascular quiver has become a routine practice. Percutaneous transluminal angioplasty (PTA) is considered a durable and safe modality for treating isolated iliac artery stenosis. Femoropopliteal angioplasty has been reported to be a success in the treatment of claudicant patients with focal lesions, although long-term outcomes are not yet satisfactory [52,53]. With availability of small vessel balloons and guide wires, infrapopliteal angioplasty is also becoming more feasible for selected cases. Recent reports indicate that PTA is feasible in most patients who have diabetes with pedal ulceration and can be effective for foot revascularization [54,55]. However, most limb salvage cases involve multilevel occlusive disease with poor distal runoff. The latter are not adequately managed with PTA at the present time. The combination of intraoperative femoral balloon angioplasty and distal bypass graft is a therapeutic strategy [56] that can afford several advantages, including preservation of saphenous vein, reduction of surgical wound, and avoidance of parallel incision at the ankle. Further progress in the techniques of brachytherapy or use of drug-eluting stents may provide further therapeutic options [57].

Summary

Findings of diminished or absent pulses, pallor on elevation, redness of the foot on lowering of the leg, sluggish refilling of the toe capillaries, and thickened nails or absence of toe hair are consistent with impaired arterial perfusion to the foot. When ischemia is recognized as contributing to pedal ulceration and infection in the diabetic foot, quantitation of its severity may be difficult. Standard clinical evaluation of trophic changes is limited in an infected foot with its accompanying swelling, edema, and erythema. A palpable pedal pulse does not preclude the possibility of the presence of limb-threatening ischemia [58]. Additional noninvasive vascular studies should be undertaken for these patients.

Management of the diabetic foot is often a complex clinical problem. However, the principles of care are simple, including correction of systemic factors, such as blood glucose control, cardiovascular risk factor management [59], and smoking [15], as well as local factor correction, such as debridement, pressure relief, infection control, and revascularization when indicated. When a patient presents with evidence of infection, adequate drainage and antibiotic therapy are mandatory. The next step should be performed to differentiate the more common neuropathic ulcerations from the truly ischemic ulceration. Symptoms of rest pain or claudication are not often helpful because many of these patients are asymptomatic as a result of the presence of their neuropathy and inactivity. If an infected foot requires debridement or open partial forefoot amputation, observing the wound on a daily base is also important. Once infection is eradicated, there should be prompt signs of healing, including the development of wound granulation within several days. If wounds are not showing signs of prompt healing, arteriography is necessary.

Early aggressive drainage, debridement, and local foot amputations combined with liberal use of revascularization results in cumulative limb salvage of 74% at 5 years in high-risk groups [60,61]. Others report that pedal bypass to the ischemic infected foot is effective and safe as long as infection adequately controlled [62]. These studies strongly suggest that early recognition and aggressive surgical drainage of pedal sepsis followed by surgical revascularization is critical to achieving maximal limb salvage in the high-risk population.

Patients who have diabetes present a unique challenge in lower extremity revascularization because of the distal origination of many bypasses, distal distribution of the occlusive disease, and the frequently calcified arterial wall. An aggressive multidisciplinary approach to foot disease associated with diabetes involving the primary care provider, medical specialists, interventional radiology, and podiatric, plastic, and vascular surgeons will provide optimal medical and surgical care. Peripheral vascular disease is highly treatable if intervention is instituted in a timely and collegial fashion.

References

[1] Sumpio BE. Foot ulcers. N Engl J Med 2000;343(11):787–93.
[2] Boulton AJ. The diabetic foot. Med Clin North Am 1988;72(6):1513–30.
[3] Knox R, Dutch W, Blume P, Sumpio BE. Diabetic foot disease. Int J Angiol 2000;9:1–6.
[4] Ebskov B, Josephsen P. Incidence of reamputation and death after gangrene of the lower extremity. Prosthet Orthot Int 1980;4(2):77–80.
[5] Kamal K, Powell RJ, Sumpio BE. The pathobiology of diabetes mellitus: implications for surgeons. J Am Coll Surg 1996;183(3):271–89.
[6] Pecoraro RE, Reiber GE, Burgess EM. Pathways to diabetic limb amputation. Basis for prevention. Diabetes Care 1990;13(5):513–21.
[7] Boulton AJ. Lawrence lecture. The diabetic foot: neuropathic in aetiology? Diabet Med 1990; 7(10):852–8.
[8] Brand FN, Abbott RD, Kannel WB. Diabetes, intermittent claudication, and risk of cardiovascular events. The Framingham Study. Diabetes 1989;38(4):504–9.
[9] Singer AJ, Clark RA. Cutaneous wound healing. N Engl J Med 1999;341(10):738–46.
[10] Akbari CM, Gibbons GW, Habershaw GM, LoGerfo FW, Veves A. The effect of arterial reconstruction on the natural history of diabetic neuropathy. Arch Surg 1997;132(2):148–52.
[11] Arora S, Pomposelli F, LoGerfo FW, Veves A. Cutaneous microcirculation in the neuropathic

diabetic foot improves significantly but not completely after successful lower extremity revascularization. J Vasc Surg 2002;35(3):501–5.
[12] Collins KA, Sumpio BE. Vascular assessment. Clin Podiatr Med Surg 2000;17(2):171–91.
[13] Abir F, Kakisis Y, Sumpio B. Do vascular surgery patients need a cardiology work-up? A review of pre-operative cardiac clearance guidelines in vascular surgery. Eur J Vasc Endovasc Surg 2003;25: 110–7.
[14] Kakisis J, Abir F, Liapis C, Sumpio B. An appraisal of different cardiac risk reduction strategies in vascular surgery patients. Eur J Vasc Endovasc Surg 2003;25:493–504.
[15] Kilaru S, Frangos SG, Chen AH, Gortler D, Dhadwal AK, Araim O, et al. Nicotine: a review of its role in atherosclerosis. J Am Coll Surg 2001;193(5):538–46.
[16] Frangos S, Kilaru S, Blume P, Shin J, Sumpio B. Classification of diabetic foot ulcers. Improving communication. Int J Angiol 2002;11:158–64.
[17] Marinelli MR, Beach KW, Glass MJ, Primozich JF, Strandness Jr DE. Noninvasive testing vs clinical evaluation of arterial disease. A prospective study. JAMA 1979;241(19):2031–4.
[18] Bone GE, Pomajzl MJ. Toe blood pressure by photoplethysmography: an index of healing in forefoot amputation. Surgery 1981;89(5):569–74.
[19] Bowers BL, Valentine RJ, Myers SI, Chervu A, Clagett GP. The natural history of patients with claudication with toe pressures of 40 mm Hg or less. J Vasc Surg 1993;18(3):506–11.
[20] Carter SA, Tate RB. Value of toe pulse waves in addition to systolic pressures in the assessment of the severity of peripheral arterial disease and critical limb ischemia. J Vasc Surg 1996;24(2): 258–65.
[21] Weitz JI, Byrne J, Clagett GP, Farkouh ME, Porter JM, Sackett DL, et al. Diagnosis and treatment of chronic arterial insufficiency of the lower extremities: a critical review. Circulation 1996;94(11): 3026–49.
[22] Gahtan V. The noninvasive vascular laboratory. Surg Clin North Am 1998;78(4):507–18.
[23] Harward TR, Volny J, Golbranson F, Bernstein EF, Fronek A. Oxygen inhalation-induced transcutaneous PO2 changes as a predictor of amputation level. J Vasc Surg 1985;2(1): 220–7.
[24] Ballard JL, Eke CC, Bunt TJ, Killeen JD. A prospective evaluation of transcutaneous oxygen measurements in the management of diabetic foot problems. J Vasc Surg 1995;22(4):485–90; discussion 90–2.
[25] Quigley FG, Faris IB. Transcutaneous oxygen tension measurements in the assessment of limb ischaemia. Clin Physiol 1991;11(4):315–20.
[26] Ligush Jr J, Reavis SW, Preisser JS, Hansen KJ. Duplex ultrasound scanning defines operative strategies for patients with limb-threatening ischemia. J Vasc Surg 1998;28(3):482–90; discussion 90–1.
[27] Wain RA, Berdejo GL, Delvalle WN, Lyon RT, Sanchez LA, Suggs WD, et al. Can duplex scan arterial mapping replace contrast arteriography as the test of choice before infrainguinal revascularization? J Vasc Surg 1999;29(1):100–7; discussion 107–9.
[28] Imparato AM, Kim GE, Madayag M, Haveson S. Angiographic criteria for successful tibial arterial reconstructions. Surgery 1973;74(6):830–8.
[29] O'Mara CS, Flinn WR, Neiman HL, Bergan JJ, Yao JS. Correlation of foot arterial anatomy with early tibial bypass patency. Surgery 1981;89(6):743–52.
[30] Berceli SA, Chan AK, Pomposelli Jr FB, Gibbons GW, Campbell DR, Akbari CM, et al. Efficacy of dorsal pedal artery bypass in limb salvage for ischemic heel ulcers. J Vasc Surg 1999; 30(3):499–508.
[31] Quader MA, Sawmiller C, Sumpio BA. Contrast-induced nephropathy: review of incidence and pathophysiology. Ann Vasc Surg 1998;12(6):612–20.
[32] Quader M, Sawmiller CJ, Sumpio BE. Radio contrast agents: history and evolution. In: J C, editor. Textbook in angiology. New York: Springer-Verlag; 2000. p. 775–83.
[33] Eisenberg RL, Bank WO, Hedgock MW. Renal failure after major angiography can be avoided with hydration. AJR Am J Roentgenol 1981;136(5):859–61.
[34] Kerstein MD, Puyau FA. Value of periangiography hydration. Surgery 1984;96(5):919–22.

[35] Rubin GD, Zarins CK. MR and spiral/helical CT imaging of lower extremity occlusive disease. Surg Clin North Am 1995;75(4):607–19.
[36] Morrison WB, Ledermann HP. Work-up of the diabetic foot. Radiol Clin North Am 2002; 40(5):1171–92.
[37] Owen RS, Baum RA, Carpenter JP, Holland GA, Cope C. Symptomatic peripheral vascular disease: selection of imaging parameters and clinical evaluation with MR angiography. Radiology 1993;187(3):627–35.
[38] Owen RS, Carpenter JP, Baum RA, Perloff LJ, Cope C. Magnetic resonance imaging of angiographically occult runoff vessels in peripheral arterial occlusive disease. N Engl J Med 1992; 326(24):1577–81.
[39] Frangos S, Kilaru S, Sumpio B, Gahtan V. Effect of gender on outcome following infrainguinal bypass graft surgery: a systematic review. Conn Med 2002;66:137–44.
[40] Frangos SG, Kilaru S, Sumpio BE, Gahtan V. Effect of gender on outcome following infrainguinal bypass graft surgery: a systematic review. Conn Med 2002;66(3):137–44.
[41] Bartlett FF, Gibbons GW, Wheelock Jr FC. Aortic reconstruction for occlusive disease. Comparable results in diabetics. Arch Surg 1986;121(10):1150–3.
[42] Brewster DC, Perler BA, Robison JG, Darling RC. Aortofemoral graft for multilevel occlusive disease. Predictors of success and need for distal bypass. Arch Surg 1982;117(12):1593–600.
[43] Steinthorsson G, Sumpio B. Clinical and biological relevance of vein cuff anastomosis. Acta Chir Belg 1999;99(6):282–8.
[44] Conrad MC. Large and small artery occlusion in diabetics and nondiabetics with severe vascular disease. Circulation 1967;36(1):83–91.
[45] Fornaini G, Leoncini G, Segni P, Fantoni A. Effect of heparin on glucose-6-phosphate dehydrogenase from normal erythrocytes and leucocytes. Ital J Biochem 1964;13(6):366–73.
[46] Plecha EJ, Seabrook GR, Bandyk DF, Towne JB. Determinants of successful peroneal artery bypass. J Vasc Surg 1993;17(1):97–105; discussion 105–6.
[47] Pomposelli Jr FB, Jepsen SJ, Gibbons GW, Campbell DR, Freeman DV, Miller A, et al. Efficacy of the dorsal pedal bypass for limb salvage in diabetic patients: short-term observations. J Vasc Surg 1990;11(6):745–51; discussion 751–2.
[48] Harrington EB, Harrington ME, Schanzer H, Jacobson JH, Haimov M. The dorsalis pedis bypass—moderate success in difficult situations. J Vasc Surg 1992;15(2):409–14; discussion 415–6.
[49] Veith FJ, Gupta SK, Samson RH, Flores SW, Janko G, Scher LA. Superficial femoral and popliteal arteries as inflow sites for distal bypasses. Surgery 1981;90(6):980–90.
[50] Mohan CR, Hoballah JJ, Martinasevic M, Chalmers RT, Sharp WJ, Kresowik TF, et al. Revascularization of the ischemic diabetic foot using popliteal artery inflow. Int Angiol 1996;15(2): 138–43.
[51] Akbari CM, Pomposelli Jr FB, Gibbons GW, Campbell DR, Pulling MC, Mydlarz D, et al. Lower extremity revascularization in diabetes: late observations. Arch Surg 2000;135(4):452–6.
[52] Hunink MG, Wong JB, Donaldson MC, Meyerovitz MF, de Vries J, Harrington DP. Revascularization for femoropopliteal disease. A decision and cost-effectiveness analysis. JAMA 1995; 274(2):165–71.
[53] Matsi PJ, Manninen HI, Vanninen RL, Suhonen MT, Oksala I, Laakso M, et al. Femoropopliteal angioplasty in patients with claudication: primary and secondary patency in 140 limbs with 1–3-year follow-up. Radiology 1994;191(3):727–33.
[54] Faglia E, Mantero M, Caminiti M, Caravagg IC, De Giglio R, Pritelli C, et al. Extensive use of peripheral angioplasty, particularly infrapopliteal, in the treatment of ischaemic diabetic foot ulcers: clinical results of a multicentric study of 221 consecutive diabetic subjects. J Intern Med 2002;252(3):225–32.
[55] Mlekusch W, Schillinger M, Sabeti S, Maca T, Ahmadi R, Minar E. Clinical outcome and prognostic factors for ischaemic ulcers treated with PTA in lower limbs. Eur J Vasc Endovasc Surg 2002;24(2):176–81.
[56] Schneider PA, Caps MT, Ogawa DY, Hayman ES. Intraoperative superficial femoral artery

balloon angioplasty and popliteal to distal bypass graft: an option for combined open and endovascular treatment of diabetic gangrene. J Vasc Surg 2001;33(5):955–62.
[57] Borromeo J, Sumpio B. Strategies in preventing intimal hyperplasia. In: Whittemore A, Bandyk D, Cronenwett J, Herrtzer N, White R, editors. Advances in vascular surgery. St. Louis (MO): Mosby; 2002. p. 201–18.
[58] Andros G, Harris RW, Dulawa LB, Oblath RW, Salles-Cunha SX. The need for arteriography in diabetic patients with gangrene and palpable foot pulses. Arch Surg 1984;119(11):1260–3.
[59] Frangos SG, Chen AH, Sumpio B. Vascular drugs in the new millennium. J Am Coll Surg 2000; 191(1):76–92.
[60] Blume P, Partagas L, Sumpio B, Attinger CE. Single stage surgical treatment of noninfected diabetic foot ulcers. J Plast Reconst Surg 2002;109:601–9.
[61] Taylor Jr LM, Porter JM. The clinical course of diabetics who require emergent foot surgery because of infection or ischemia. J Vasc Surg 1987;6(5):454–9.
[62] Tannenbaum GA, Pomposelli Jr FB, Marcaccio EJ, Gibbons GW, Campbell DR, Freeman DV, et al. Safety of vein bypass grafting to the dorsal pedal artery in diabetic patients with foot infections. J Vasc Surg 1992;15(6):982–8; discussion 989–90.

CLINICS IN PODIATRIC MEDICINE AND SURGERY

Clin Podiatr Med Surg 20 (2003) 709–728

Diabetic foot ulcerations: management and adjunctive therapy

Robert G. Frykberg, DPM, MPH

Carl T. Hayden VA Medical Center, 650 East Indian School Road, Phoenix, AZ 85012, USA

The most significant of all foot lesions in the diabetic patient is an ulceration, often referred to as a mal perforans ulcer. Whether of neuropathic or ischemic origin, a diabetic foot ulcer is potentially limb threatening. Its presence places the foot at high risk for progressing to the more serious complications of sepsis, gangrene, and subsequent amputation. The final outcome is therefore dependent upon multiple factors, all of which relate to the appropriateness of therapy and the time at which it is instituted.

The "diabetic foot syndrome" and attendant sequelae account for direct medical expenditures of hundreds of millions of dollars annually, long hospital stays, and lengthy periods of disability [1–3]. Of the estimated 17 million persons in the United States with diabetes mellitus, approximately 15% to 20% will be hospitalized with a foot complication at some time during the course of their disease [4,5]. Unfortunately, many of these patients will require lower extremity amputation at some level as a consequence of fulminating infection or peripheral ischemia, in concert with neuropathy as a predisposing factor.

Foot ulceration is recognized as one of the major risk factors for amputation [6–8]. Although the triad of neuropathy, deformity, and trauma are frequent component causes in its pathogenesis, the diabetic foot ulcer can further be attributed to numerous other important risk factors [9–13]. Early detection of these risk factors as well as of foot ulcers themselves are key components in the overall management of diabetic foot disorders and amputation prevention programs [14]. Prompt and aggressive treatment of diabetic foot ulcers can often prevent an exacerbation of the problem and the potential need for amputation. The aim of therapy, therefore, should be early intervention to allow prompt healing of the lesion, and once healed, to prevent its recurrence. As will be discussed, optimal care for foot ulceration depends upon the treating physicians' understanding of the

E-mail address: robert.frykberg@med.va.gov

doi:10.1016/S0891-8422(03)00069-7

pathophysiology involved, familiarity with accepted principles of treatment, and the knowledge that a coordinated multidisciplinary team approach will best accomplish the goal of limb salvage. Above all else, prevention of foot lesions should be the ultimate aim [14,15].

Epidemiology

Several population-based studies report an annual incidence of diabetic foot ulceration in the range of 2% to 3% in IDDM and NIDDM patients, whereas the prevalence varies between 4% and 10% (see references [13,16–18]). These studies also indicate a general trend for higher frequencies of ulceration with increasing age and duration of diabetes. A 3-year retrospective cohort study of 8905 patients in a large health maintenance organization who have diabetes reported a 5.8% cumulative incidence of ulceration (approximately 2% per year) [18]. In the largest prospective study reported to date, 219 of 6613 patients who have diabetes from the United Kingdom developed foot ulceration over a 2-year period (2.2% average annual incidence) [13]. The consistency of these data suggests the reliability of these estimates. Unfortunately, once sustaining an ulceration, recurrence rates can reach 50% at 2 years and 70% at 5 years [8].

Patients who have diabetic foot ulcers have also been determined to have an increased risk for mortality when compared with nonulcerated counterparts [18–20]. Boyko [19] reported a 2.4-fold risk of death in patients who have diabetic ulcers after adjustment for age, duration, glucose control, amputation, and smoking history. Ramsey, in a 1999 retrospective cohort study of 8905 patients with diabetes [18], reported a 3-year survival of only 72% in those with foot ulcers versus 87% in age and sex-matched nonulcerated patients. In a recent single-prospective cohort study of patients with new diabetic foot ulcers, the 5-year mortality rate was 44%, although there was no reported comparison with nonulcerated cohorts [20]. Mortality was highest (55%) in those patients who had ischemic ulcers.

Amputation is one of the more prevalent major complications of diabetes mellitus, accounting for 86,000 diabetes-related discharges in 1996 [3]. Approximately 80% to 85% of lower extremity amputations (LEA) are preceded by foot ulceration [6,21]. Furthermore, after adjusting for numerous other confounders, several prospective studies have confirmed the independent risk that foot ulcers confer toward amputation in patients who have diabetes, with relative risks in the range of 2.5% to 3.2% [7,16]. In cohorts of patients developing ulcers, approximately 12% to 19% require LEA within 3 to 5 years (see references [8,18,20]). Tragically, the 3-year survival rate after one major lower extremity amputation is only 50%, whereas the 5-year survival is only about 40% [22,23]. In addition, 50% of those patients undergoing an LEA of one limb will develop a serious contralateral lesion within 2 years, thereby placing the fate of the second limb in jeopardy as well [8,24].

Etiologies

Multiple factors involving intrinsic complications of diabetes mellitus in concert with various extrinsic forces or risk factors place the diabetic patient at particularly high risk for lower extremity lesions [10–13]. The triad of peripheral neuropathy, deformity, and minor trauma has emerged as the most frequent component causes in the possible causal pathways leading to foot ulceration [9]. Though neuropathy, trauma, and deformity were present in 78%, 77%, and 63% of 32 unique causal pathways to ulcer in this study of 148 patients, peripheral ischemia (35%), edema (37%), and callus (30%) were also frequently represented. Infection was a precursor to ulceration in only 1% of their cases.

Peripheral sensory neuropathy as measured by Vibration Perception Thresholds (VPT) can impart a 3.4- to 32-fold risk of ulceration [25–28]. Insensitivity to a 10-g monofilament, commonly used to assess peripheral neuropathy, has been shown in several studies to convey a 2.2- to18-fold risk of ulceration (see references [11,25,26,29]). In the large population-based North-West Diabetes Foot Care Study, loss of protective sensation (LOPS) to the 10-g monofilament increased the risk of ulceration by 80%; abnormal ankle reflexes increased this risk by 55% [13].

Impaired cutaneous circulation and peripheral arterial disease are also major risk factors for ulceration and LEA (see references [6,7,9,11,14]). Transcutaneous oxygen tension ($TcPO_2$) levels less than 30 mmHg and absence of peripheral pulses or history of previous revascularization are each strong independent predictors of ulceration (see references [11,29,30]), whereas TcPO2 less than 20 mmHg can result in a 39-fold increased risk of ulcer wound healing failure [31]. Doppler ankle systolic pressures and ankle/brachial indices (ABI) are frequently elevated in patients who have diabetes because of medial arterial calcification. This false elevation of arterial pressures confounds the usefulness of such testing in the prediction of ulceration and healing. Therefore, toe systolic pressures might be more reliable measures of arterial perfusion in this regard (see references [30,32,33]). Diabetic foot infections frequently develop in and complicate established foot ulcers. Whereas infection is a major component in the pathway to lower limb amputation, susceptibility to infection plays a minor role in the causation of ulceration [6,9].

Although most ulcers are initially precipitated by chronic or acute trauma (extrinsic factors) (see references [6,9,34]), numerous additional intrinsic contributory factors might predispose the patient who has diabetes to develop foot lesions (Box 1) [10–12,35]. Prior history of ulceration or amputation, age, weight, duration of diabetes, nephropathy, retinopathy, limited joint mobility, high plantar pressures, and structural deformity (ie, Charcot foot) have all been implicated as putative risk factors for ulceration (see references [11,14,25,32]). Faulty biomechanical function often results from these complications of diabetes and predisposes the foot to injury as well (see references [34,36,37]). Neuropathy-induced muscle imbalance, including anterior crural and intrinsic muscle weakness, gastrocnemius equinus, osteoarthropathy, partial foot amputations, and

Box 1. Risk factors for ulceration

- Neuropathy
  - Sensory
  - Motor
  - Autonomic
- Deformity (hammertoes, Charcot)
- Minor Trauma
  - High plantar pressures
  - Shoe pressure
  - High impact
- Improper foot care
- Thermal injury
  - Hot soaks
  - Frostbite
- Limited joint mobility
- Vascular disease
  - Macrovascular (ischemia)
  - Microvascular (impaired thermoregulation)
- Previous ulceration
- Amputation
- Nephropathy
- Age
- Duration of diabetes
- Blindness
- Hyperglycemia
- Cigarette smoking

associated gait abnormalities, contribute to the abnormal loading patterns and high pressure areas characteristic of the neuropathic diabetic foot [37,38].

Evaluation

A thorough and systematic lower extremity examination is indispensable when initiating treatment of a diabetic foot ulcer (see references [5,12,14]). Before the physical examination, however, it is important to inspect the shoes for appropriate fit, foreign objects, and wear patterns. The clinical evaluation must include an assessment of the ulcer's etiology, its size and depth, presence of local and systemic infection, and peripheral vascular status [5,12]. An evaluation of the patient's general health and diabetes control, a quantification of peripheral neuropathy, and a thorough dermatologic and musculoskeletal examination must also be performed.

Bilateral lower extremity pulses should be palpated. When dorsalis pedis or posterior tibial pulses are absent or diminished, Doppler segmental pressures to the toes or $TcPO_2$ evaluation is indicated and vascular consultation should be sought [5,14]. Arteriography is frequently necessary and, in the pulseless foot, is sometimes recommended in lieu of noninvasive testing [34].

The neurological examination should evaluate the patient's sensory perception, muscle strength, and deep tendon reflexes. Ankle and knee reflexes are easily assessed with a neurological hammer. The key elements in evaluating sensitivity are impaired sensation to pain, light touch, and hot/cold and vibratory sensation. Pain perception is easily evaluated by testing with a disposable needle. A cotton ball, lamb's wool, or 10-g monofilament may be used to assess light touch, and a 128 Hz tuning fork or biothesiometer (Biomedical, Newbury, OH) are recommended for vibratory evaluation. Inability to perceive a 10-g (5.07) Semmes-Weinstein monofilament is indicative of peripheral neuropathy, as is VPT greater than 25 [25–28]. Both correlate well with risk for ulceration as previously outlined. Cold perception is easily evaluated by submerging the metal handle of one's neurological hammer into cold water and then placing it against the patient's skin. Autonomic neuropathy, widely prevalent in patients with ulcers or peripheral sensory neuropathy, can be recognized by anhidrotic skin with cracks or fissures. Diagnostic modalities for autonomic dysfunction, such as QSART for sudomotor function or cardiac autonomic function testing, are available but infrequently employed in most clinical settings.

Structural deformities, such as hammertoes, previous partial foot amputation, or Charcot neuroarthropathy, frequently create high pressure areas that result in ulceration (see references ([9,14,34,36,39]. The musculoskeletal evaluation should not only involve a visual inspection for such findings, but also test for muscle strength, weakness (foot drop, intrinsic muscle atrophy), and contractures (gastocnemius equinus). Assessment of joint range of motion and gait evaluation with computerized plantar pressure analysis will also be of help in fully understanding the abnormal dysfunction contributing to ulceration [26]. Abnormally high plantar pressure areas, often clinically evident from callus, erythema, or warmth even in the absence of ulceration, can be identified and quantified with several types of force or pressure measurement systems (see references [37,40,41]). In-shoe devices with thin pressure sensors and force plate or pressure mat computerized systems are in fairly common use despite their expense and time requirements and have helped to ascertain the significant role that such pressures play in the pathogenesis of ulceration (see references [25,26,41]). Less expensive, noncomputerized footprint pressure-mapping devices have also become commercially available to the practitioner for rapid pressure assessment, which can become a permanent part of the patient's record [42].

The dermatologic examination should assess the skin and interdigital areas of both feet with particular attention to skin quality and integrity, atrophy, and callus formation as well as other ulcerative or preulcerative changes. Skin color changes in association with petechial rashes, small eschars, or heel fissures might indicate a critical level of ischemia. Toenail changes and the presence of subungual drainage or paronychiae might frequently be a source of more proximal infection. Thickened or dystrophic onychomycotic toenails can potentially cause subungual pressure ulceration. Close inspection of such nail pathology, especially when loosened from the nail bed, might reveal otherwise unrecognized lesions [43].

Wound assessment

Clinical evaluation of the wound should include a description of its appearance and measurement of the ulcer's dimensions (Box 2) [5]. A tracing of the ulcer on a transparent film or plastic sheet can facilitate this process. This should be recorded and remeasured at subsequent visits to evaluate treatment progress. Digital close-up photography also aids in this regard and can be appropriately incorporated into the patient's chart or electronic medical record. The depth and extent of the wound should be explored with a small, sterile, blunt probe. Particular care must be taken to probe for hidden sinus tracts and deep abscesses as well as to identify tendon, muscle, bone, and joint involvement. Palpable bone in the depths of diabetic pedal ulcers is strongly correlated with osteomyelitis [44].

Clinical signs of infection, such as purulent drainage, odor, cellulitis, fever, and leukocytosis, must be recorded, although the latter two might not always be evident even in the presence of osteomyelitis [45–47]. Aerobic and anaerobic cultures should be obtained from curettage of the ulcer base because this method has proven more reliable in elucidating the true underlying pathogens [46,48]. Radiological evaluation is necessary to ascertain the presence of osteomyelitis, recognizing that radiographs have a low sensitivity and should not be solely relied upon in determining the need for further interventions [49,50]. As indicated, other imaging modalities can aid in the diagnosis of osteomyelitis. Technetium bone

Box 2. Wound assessment

1. Wound description (color, slough, necrotic tissue)
2. Wound dimensions (size, area, depth)
3. Probe for depth, bone, sinus tracts
4. Determine presence of infection
   a. Cultures as indicated
5. Assess for neuropathy
   a. Monofilaments, vibrations, two-point discrimination
6. Vascularity
   a. Pulses, rubor, temperature
   b. Noninvasive tests
      1. ABI, Doppler waveforms, TcPO2
      2. Angiography
7. Determine etiology
8. Classification
   a. Grade, neuropathic, ischemic, neuroischemic

scans, indium, and Tc-99m HMPAO-labeled leukocyte scans, monoclonal antigranulocyte antibody scans, CT scans, and MRI are all useful in this regard, each having their own strengths and limitations [51–55]. However, the value of these expensive imaging tests has been questioned in terms of improved outcomes above those achieved with empirical surgical and medical therapy [56]. A rational approach to the use of these modalities in concert with a careful clinical examination can optimize patient care by early recognition or exclusion of underlying bone infection.

Classification of ulcerations can facilitate a logical approach to treatment and aid in the prediction of healing outcomes [5]. Several wound classification systems have been offered based on such parameters as extent of infection, neuropathy, ischemia, depth or extent of tissue loss, or location [57–61]. The most widely accepted classification system for diabetic foot ulcers and lesions is the one proposed by Wagner that is based upon the depth of penetration and extent of tissue necrosis [58]. In this system, the various lesions found in the diabetic foot are separated into six categories or grades from 0 to 5. However, it does not specifically address neuropathy, ischemia, or infection. Recognizing such shortcomings, the University of Texas Classification System specifically addresses the significant role that infection and ischemia play in the outcome of such lesions (Table 1) [59]. This scheme has been validated to show that increasingly more severe categories of wounds have poorer outcomes and higher rates of amputation [59,60]. Although no clinically useful system can fully describe all facets of a diabetic foot ulcer, appropriate wound assessment should include wound dimensions, tissue level involved, and associated attributes as well as consideration of host and environmental factors.

Treatment

Management of the foot ulcer is dictated by such parameters as acuity, its severity, extent of tissue loss (grade), ischemia, and presence of infection [12]. A systematic approach to treatment should be taken for all diabetic foot lesions that addresses each of the basic tenets indicated in Box 3. A multidisciplinary team approach should be employed because of the multifaceted nature of the disease itself and for managing the numerous comorbidities attendant with foot ulceration

Table 1
University of Texas wound classification system

	Grade			
Stage	0	1	2	3
A	Pre- or postulcerative lesion (epithelialized)	Superficial not involving tendon, capsule or bone	Penetrates to tendon or capsule	Penetrates to Bone
B	Infection	Infection	Infection	Infection
C	Ischemia	Ischemia	Ischemia	Ischemia
D	Infection and ischemia	Infection and ischemia	Infection and ischemia	Infection and ischemia

Box 3. Alternative wound-healing modalities

Vacuum-assisted closure (VAC)
Noncontact normothermic wound therapy (NNWT)
Hyperbaric oxygen (HBO)
Electrical stimulation
Medicinal larvae therapy (MLT)
Bioengineered tissue substitutes
Growth factors

[15,34]. This approach has resulted in significant improvements in outcomes, such as faster healing, decreased times to healing or lengths of hospital stay, and reductions in the incidence of major amputation (see references [21,62–65]).

Thorough assessment of the patient and wound should facilitate treatment by appropriately addressing those parameters found in the course of the examination. The wound should be classified and, accordingly, the degree of acuity or severity will determine the need for hospitalization or surgical intervention. For instance, a superficial, noninfected neuropathic ulcer with easily palpable pedal pulses would most often be treated in an outpatient setting. In contrast, an ischemic wound with obvious infection, deep abscess, and suspected osteomyelitis should be hospitalized for thorough work-up, vascular consultation, and aggressive surgical and medical management [14].

Management of hyperglycemia, ketoacidosis, renal insufficiency, and the numerous other comorbidities that might coexist in the ulcerated patient must be addressed concurrently with management of the foot lesion. Internal medicine, endocrinology, and cardiology consultations are frequently required for managing the acutely infected patient who requires urgent hospitalization. Such consultations should be sought early in the course of treatment to optimize metabolic control, even when non–limb-threatening lesions are treated in the ambulatory setting.

Wound care is best facilitated by sharp debridement of callus, fibrotic, and necrotic tissue back to a bleeding base (see references [5,14,66,67]). Topical enzymes have not been proven as effective in this regard, although there has been a resurgent interest in papain-urea and collagenase products, which provide "maintenance debridement" after initial sharp debridement between office visits [68,69]. Biosurgical debridement (larva therapy) with medical sterile maggots has also seen increased use in recent years after falling into disfavor with the advent of modern antibiotic therapies. Though several case series and reviews document the potential usefulness of medicinal larva therapy for difficult diabetic foot wounds, clinical trials are still lacking [70,71].

Soaking diabetic foot lesions should be avoided because these insensitive or ischemic feet can easily be scalded by hot water. Although there are numerous types of topical medications, gels, and antiseptics (ie, povidone-iodine) promoted for ulcer care, few have proven more efficacious than saline wet dressings, which are still considered the gold standard to which new agents are compared (see references [5,14,72]). A warm, moist environment that is protected from external contamination is most conducive to wound healing [72,73]. Modern dressings integrate not only the moist wound-healing concept, but also those of exudate or protease management, topical antibacterial activity, and autolytic debridement. These attributes can variably be provided by a number of commercially available special dressings, including semipermeable films, hydrocolloids, polyurethane foams, silver-coated dressings, hyaluronic acid fibers, oxidized regenerated cellulose, and calcium alginates (see references [66,72,73]). There has also been an interest in collagen-based wound-healing products or dressings as possible donors of this protein for incorporation into the healing wound extracellular matrix or to provide a framework for ingrowth of new tissue [66,74]. One such product, Oasis (Cook Biomedical/Healthpoint, West Lafayette, Indiana), is actually an acellular collagen xenograft derived from porcine small intestinal submucosa (SIS) [75]. Although currently undergoing clinical trials, this sterile collagen dressing has shown early promise in expediting wound repair when used in conjunction with other overlying secondary dressings for exudate and moisture management [76]. Unfortunately, most of the aforementioned wound-healing agents or dressings have been marketed without the benefit of randomized controlled clinical trials to demonstrate their efficacy or superiority over standard therapy (moist dressings) in achieving complete wound healing. Since the 1999 Consensus Development Conference on diabetic foot wound care, there has been a plea to base the adoption of new technologies and products on scientific evidence to support their usefulness [5,66]. Though much of wound care is still based on art rather than science or evidence, the expense of these new technologies is a compelling reason for practitioners to preferentially use those agents, devices, or products that have documented efficacy in expediting wound repair.

The role of growth factors as adjunctive agents in promoting wound repair is under intense investigation, although only one commercially available product is available for widespread use (see references [66,72,77]). These agents stimulate chemotaxis and mitogenesis of neutrophils, fibroblasts, and monocytes as well as other components that form the cellular basis of wound healing. Becaplermin, a topically applied platelet-derived growth factor gel (Regranex, Ethicon (a division of Johnson & Johnson, Somerville, New Jersey) is approved for use on neuropathic diabetic foot ulcers. In concert with appropriate debridement and off-loading, becaplermin has been shown to provide a 43% increase in complete healing within 20 weeks as compared with standard therapy with placebo gel and saline dressings [78].

Tissue-engineered human dermis (Dermagraft, Advanced Tissue Sciences, La Jolla, California) or living skin equivalent (Apligraf, Novartis Pharmaceuticals, East Hanover, New Jersey) are fairly recent types of tissue implants approved for diabetic foot ulcers that have proven efficacy for expediting wound healing when compared with standard therapy with saline dressings [79,80]. These bioengineered implants, consisting of cultured neonatal fibroblasts, are living tissues that act as donors of growth factors and secrete extracellular matrix components into the host wound bed. Both tissue substitutes have received FDA approval for treating diabetic foot ulcers, having shown by clinical trials to significantly expedite complete wound healing of foot ulcers in comparison to saline dressings after 12 weeks. As always, these and any other agents or modalities cannot supplant attention to the basic tenets of wound care, including adequate debridement and off-loading [5,14].

A fairly new technology that is gaining widespread acceptance in the management of deep diabetic foot wounds or open amputation sites is vacuum-assisted closure (VAC, Kinetic Concepts, San Antonio, Texas) using negative pressure therapy [81]. Although formal clinical trials are being conducted, anecdotal and retrospective studies indicate that this therapy is useful in managing open wounds by controlling exudates and stimulating the formation of a granular tissue bed [82,83]. As part of multimodal therapy for such wounds, vacuum-assisted closure can prepare wounds for grafting, tissue substitutes, or delayed closure. Alternatively, this modality can be used as the sole therapy employed to promote healing by secondary intention after appropriate debridement and management of infection.

Noncontact normothermic wound therapy (NNWT) is another modality currently undergoing clinical trials for diabetic foot wounds (Warm-UP; Augustine Medical, Eden Prairie, Minnesota) [84,85]. Based on the principles of warm, moist wound healing, NNWT contains a heating element incorporated into a noncontact, semiocclusive, moisture-retentive dressing administered three times daily. Theoretically, wound repair is enhanced as the surface warming increases blood flow and oxygen tension to the area under the closed system. A recent preliminary report of an ongoing trial of NNWR compared with saline-moistened gauze noted a trend for increased healing in the NNWT group but did not reach statistical significance because of an inadequate sample size [84].

Pressure relief

Appropriate relief of pressure and off-loading the wound should be initiated at first presentation. Ill-fitting footwear should be discarded and replaced with a surgical sandal, wedged surgical shoe, or other type of temporary footwear that can accomplish the goal of removing pressure from the foot ulcer (see references [12,86,87]). When the lesion is on the dorsum of a toe or on either side of the foot, a simple cutout can be made in the patient's shoe. If total non–weightbearing with crutches is not feasible, a pressure-attenuating felt, foam, or plastazote insert should be used in the surgical shoe [88]. However, the total-contact cast (TCC) is considered the optimal method to protect the nonischemic ulceration during ambulation by virtue of its ability to redistribute high pressures from under the ulcer to the entire foot and leg encompassed by the cylindrical cast (see references [34,87,89–91]). Acceptable alternatives to the TCC are the Scotchcast Boot or removable walking braces [87,92]. However, any removable device raises the concern for patient noncompliance with the prescribed off-loading therapy.

Infection

Most severe diabetic foot infections are polymicrobial, although this is not routinely true for mild or non–limb-threatening infections wherein a single isolate might be recovered (see references [48,49,93]). Wounds that do not appear to be clinically infected and have no purulent drainage or cellulitis generally do not need to be cultured because they can be expected to have colonizing flora that do not require antimicrobial therapy [48]. Conversely, ulcers demonstrating such classic signs of infection are best cultured from a curettage or biopsy of the ulcer base [93]. However, recent reports indicate that a swab culture of the wound or purulent secretions are fairly concordant with tissue specimens and can therefore guide antibiotic therapy appropriately [94]. Treatment should be initiated with broad spectrum antibiotics after first obtaining reliable aerobic and anaerobic cultures [14]. Therapy should subsequently be tailored according to the clinical response of the patient and results of culture and sensitivity testing. Intravenous or oral agents can be used, often in combination, depending on the severity of infection and isolates recovered (see references [46,48,49,95]). Surgical drainage and deep debridement of soft tissue and bone or local partial amputation are necessary adjuncts to antibiotic therapy (see references [34,47,96]). Underlying osteomyelitis is frequently present in moderate to severe infections and requires aggressive bony resection of infected bone and joints followed by 4 to 6 weeks of culture-directed antibiotics (see references [14,47,50,97]).

Ischemia

Treatment of underlying ischemia is critical in achieving a successful outcome. Vascular surgical consultation should be obtained upon presentation of an ischemic wound and in cases where ulcers show no sign of progress despite appropriate management. Extreme distal arterial reconstruction to restore pulsatile flow to the foot is a major component of the limb salvage strategy in such patients [33,98]. The role of isolated endovascular procedures is still to be determined, although such interventions are frequently performed in concert with angiography preceding vascular reconstructive procedures [34,99].

Hyperbaric oxygen therapy (HBOT) has been used for adjunctive treatment of foot ulcers in an attempt to hyperoxygenate the skin and soft tissues [100,101]. Benefits of HBO therapy, in addition to increasing blood oxygen content, include edema reduction, granulation tissue formation, enhanced collagen production, and enhanced bacterial killing by leukocytes [101]. However, this modality still suffers from a paucity of carefully controlled clinical trials [5,102]. There are several reviews and retrospective and prospective studies on this modality that purport efficacy in difficult wounds where there might be nonreconstructable occlusive vascular disease or limb-threatening infection [100–102]. Local, topically applied oxygen has not been proven effective and cannot be advocated for use [103]. HBO and other alternative technologies that might be used in the management of diabetic foot wounds are listed in Box 3. Confidence in their ability to effectively aid in the healing of diabetic foot wounds, however, should be reserved until such technologies have been subjected to randomized, controlled clinical trials [5,66].

Surgical management

Surgical management of diabetic foot ulcers plays a key role not only in eradicating indolent sites of infection but in removing or correcting bony deformities that contribute to the pathogenesis of the ulcer (see references [14,104,105]). Once considered ill-advised, curative or prophylactic foot surgery is now recognized as an important facet of amputation prevention programs (see references [5,15,34,106]). The incorporation of a surgical approach to foot ulcer management has met with improved outcomes, faster healing times, and fewer recurrences with acceptable frequencies of postoperative complications [106–111]. Others report a preference for surgical therapy over total-contact casting to avoid secondary cast lesions and to remove underlying bony prominences that might result in ulcer recurrence [112].

Surgical intervention can generally be classified as curative, ablative, or elective [14,104]. A modification of this scheme based on level of risk or acuity in the presence of a limb-threatening infection has been proposed wherein a fourth class (emergent) is added that can encompass any type of ablative or curative procedure that is used for urgent limb salvage [105].

Curative surgery is performed in the presence of a nonhealing ulcer or a chronically recurring one when off-loading and standard wound care techniques are not effective [14,104]. Various surgical procedures have been described in the literature that are employed to remove areas of chronically increased peak pressure, usually over structural deformities (see references [43,104,113,114]). Such procedures also include resections of infected bone or joints as an alternative to partial foot amputation (see references [108,112,115]). Operations frequently performed in this regard might include exostectomy, digital arthroplasty, sesamoidectomy, single or multiple metatarsal head resections, joint resections, tendo-Achilles lengthening, or partial calcanectomy (see references [104,108,116,117]). Various plastic surgical techniques including local flaps, free flaps, and skin grafts can also be effectively used for managing such lesions [111,118]. A recent study using single-stage ulcer and bone excision with local flap coverage has shown a 97% healing rate in a median time of 31 days [111].

Ablative surgery, usually synonymous with amputation, is a common sequela to gangrene, infections, and ulcers associated with osteomyelitis. Such procedures are frequently performed on an emergent basis for acute limb-threatening infection and might include open or guillotine amputations [119]. Foot-sparing amputations commonly include lesser and great toe, first ray, lesser rays, and transmetatarsal or midfoot amputations (see references [108,119,120]). Subtotal or partial calcanectomy might also be considered in this regard as a hindfoot amputation. This procedure has seen increased usage in recent years because it can effectively preserve limbs previously destined for amputation [115,116]. Symes amputations are also considered limb salvaging because they are performed at the ankle level, although they are not as frequently performed because of prosthetic-fitting difficulties [119]. Ablative surgical intervention requires removal of all infected and necrotic tissue to the level of viable soft tissue and bone. Optimally, such procedures are performed in a manner that allows for the maximum function from the remaining portion of the limb [14,34].

Primary wound closure is suitable if no infection or ischemic tissue remains and enough soft tissue is available [14]. In the presence of marginal ischemia, a primary closure is always preferred. Secondary wound healing with or without adjunctive wound therapies may still be the best choice for some patients. Wounds may be packed open initially, requiring well-controlled and frequently assessed wound care with delayed primary closure or closure by secondary intention [112]. Open wounds, including amputation sites, can also be managed with subatmospheric negative-pressure dressings until ready for definitive closure or until closed by secondary intention [82]. There has also been success reported with primary closure of marginally infected wounds over a closed antibiotic instillation system or over antibiotic-impregnated beads [121,122]. Mechanical assistance using various skin stretching devices are the surgeon's option and may help to attain delayed primary closure for some wounds [123]. Plastic surgical techniques as previously discussed are other options that may be used [111]. All patients must be assessed on an individual basis for the selection of the surgical management that best meets their needs.

Many of the procedures previously mentioned in the discussion on curative surgery would also be indicated in the elective reconstruction of the nonulcerated foot. Patients requiring prophylactic or elective surgery might simply be at risk of ulceration by virtue of peripheral neuropathy or prior history of ulceration. Surgical correction of structural deformities in the carefully selected patient can serve to reduce high-pressure areas that cannot be accommodated by therapeutic footwear (see references [5,34,57,104]). Common operations performed in this regard include the correction of hammertoes, bunions, prominent metatarsal heads, exostectomies, and tendo-Achilles lengthening [43,115,117]. Proper patient selection and evaluation is extremely important before performing elective surgery in these high-risk patients. Patients' general medical and diabetes status should be optimal and their cardiovascular status must be stable enough to undergo an anesthetic session. Therefore, local or regional anesthesia with sedation is usually recommended, especially in those patients with significant peripheral neuropathy. Peripheral vascular disease must be recognized as an impediment to successful healing and, when present, appropriately addressed with operative or endovascular revascularization before prophylactic surgery [33,34].

The basic guidelines or tenets for the management of diabetic foot ulcers are summarized in Box 4.

Prevention

A multidisciplinary team approach focused on prevention of new or recurrent foot lesions and amputations has been shown to be the most successful way to manage high-risk patients [21,62–65]. Such teams, variably consisting of a podiatrist/podiatric surgeon, internist, endocrinologist, infectious disease special-

Box 4. Basic tenets for treatment of diabetic foot ulcers

Rest and pressure reduction
- Crutch, wheelchair, contact cast, cast brace, off-loading surgical shoe

Medical treatment
- Hyperglycemia, hypertension, electrolyte imbalance, renal insufficiency

Infection
- Incision and drainage, culture, antibiotics, bone and joint resections, amputations

Vascular
- Distal bypass to foot; restore pulsatile flow

Wound care
- Debridement, topical saline or cleansers, growth factors, special dressings, HBO
- Prophylactic surgery (curative, ablative, reconstructive)

ist, vascular surgeon, orthopedic surgeon, teaching nurse, and pedorthist have subsequently reported dramatic reductions in rates of lower extremity amputations and improved ulceration healing rates [63,64]. A key facet of prevention is patient and provider education (see references [5,14,15,124]). Patients must learn the importance of daily foot inspection, proper foot care, early intervention, and recognition of risk factors for diabetic foot disorders. Regular podiatric visits, including debridement of calluses and ingrown toenails, provide an opportunity to reinforce appropriate self-care behavior and allow for early detection of new or impending foot problems [14,15]. Providers need to be kept abreast of current diagnostic techniques, risk factor assessment, and treatment guidelines [124]. Therapeutic shoes with pressure-relieving insoles, rocker soles, and high toe boxes that protect the high-risk foot are an essential element of the prevention program and have been associated with significant reductions in ulcer development (see references [34,62,125,126]). A recent clinical trial of therapeutic shoes in a mixed group of non–high-risk patients who have diabetes without significant deformity found no significant protection afforded by custom therapeutic shoes and insoles [127]. Because of a number of methodological concerns, these results most appropriately should not be generalized to high-risk individuals with neuropathy and deformity [128].

Summary

Foot ulcerations, infections, gangrene, and lower extremity amputation are major causes of disability to the patient who has diabetes mellitus, often resulting in significant morbidity, extensive periods of hospitalization, and mortality. Although not all such lesions can be prevented, it is possible to dramatically reduce their incidence through appropriate management and prevention protocols incorporating a multidisciplinary team approach.

References

[1] Centers for Disease Control and Prevention. Diabetes: a serious public health problem. At a glance 2000. Washington, DC: US Department of Health and Human Services; 2000.

[2] Reiber GE, Boyko EJ, Smith DG. Lower extremity foot ulcers and amputations in diabetes. In: Harris MI, Cowie C, Stern MP, editors. Diabetes in America. 2nd edition. Bethesda (MD): National Institutes of Health; 1995. Publication #NIH 95–1468. p. 409–28.

[3] Centers for Disease Control and Prevention. Diabetes surveillance, 1999. US Department of Health and Human Services. Available at: http://www.cdc.gov/diabetes/statistics/surv199/chap6/chapter6Intro.htm. Accessed March 10, 2003.

[4] American Diabetes Association. Facts and figures. Available at: http://www.diabetes.org/main/info/facts/facts.jsp. Accessed March 10, 2003.

[5] American Diabetes Association. Consensus Development Conference on diabetic foot wound care. Diabetes Care 1999;22:1354–60.

[6] Pecoraro RE, Reiber G, Burgess EM. Pathways to diabetic limb amputation: basis for prevention. Diabetes Care 1990;13:513–21.

[7] Adler AI, Boyko EJ, Ahroni J, Smith DG. Lower-extremity amputation in diabetes: the independent effects of peripheral vascular disease, sensory neuropathy, and foot ulcers. Diabetes Care 1999;22:1029–35.

[8] Apelquist J, Larsson J, Agardh C-D. Long term prognosis for patients with foot ulcers. J Int Med 1993;233:485–91.

[9] Reiber GE, Vileikyte L, Boyko EJ, et al. Causal pathways for incident lower-extremity ulcers in patients with diabetes from two settings. Diabetes Care 1999;22:157–62.

[10] Abbott CA, Vileikyte L, Williamson S, et al. Multicenter study of the incidence and predictive risk factors for diabetic neuropathic foot ulceration. Diabetes Care 1998;21:1071–5.

[11] Boyko EJ, Ahroni JH, Stensel V, et al. A prospective study of risk factors for diabetic foot ulcer: the Seattle Diabetic Foot Study. Diabetes Care 1999;22:1036–42.

[12] Frykberg RG. Diabetic foot ulcers: pathogenesis and management. Am Fam Physician 2002;66:1655–62.

[13] Abbott CA, Carrington AL, Ashe H, et al. The North-West Diabetes Foot Care Study: incidence of, and risk factors for, new diabetic foot ulceration in a community-based patient cohort. Diabetic Med 2002;19:377–84.

[14] Frykberg RG, Armstrong DG, Giurini J, et al. Diabetic foot disorders: a clinical practice guideline. J Foot Ankle Surg 2000;39(Suppl 1):2–60.

[15] Frykberg RG. Team approach toward lower extremity amputation prevention in diabetes. J Am Pod Med Assoc 1997;87:305–12.

[16] Moss S, Klein R, Klein B. The 14-year incidence of lower extremity amputations in a diabetic population: the Wisconsin Epidemiologic Study of Diabetic Retinopathy. Diabetes Care 1999;22:951–9.

[17] Kumar S, Ashe HA, Parnell LN, et al. The prevalence of foot ulceration and its correlates in type 2 diabetic patients: a population-based study. Diabetic Med 1994;11:480–4.

[18] Ramsey SD, Newton K, Blough D, et al. Incidence, outcomes, and cost of foot ulcers in patients with diabetes. Diabetes Care 1999;22:382–7.

[19] Boyko EJ, Ahroni JH, Smith DG, Davignon D. Increased mortality associated with diabetic foot ulcer. Diabet Med 1996;13:967–72.

[20] Moulik PK, Mtonga R, Gill GV. Amputation and mortality in new-onset diabetic foot ulcers stratified by etiology. Diabetes Care 2003;26:491–4.

[21] Larsson J, Apelqvist J, Agardh C-D, Stenstrom A. Decreasing incidence of major amputation in diabetic patients: a consequence of a multidisciplinary foot care team approach? Diabetic Med 1995;12:770–6.
[22] American Diabetes Association. Diabetes 1996 vital statistics. Alexandria (VA): American Diabetes Association; 1996.
[23] Lee JS, Lu M, Lee VS, et al. Lower-extremity amputation: incidence, risk factors, and mortality in the Oklahoma Indian Diabetes Study. Diabetes 1993;42:876–82.
[24] Goldner MG. The fate of the second leg in the diabetic amputee. Diabetes 1960;9:100–3.
[25] Pham H, Armstrong DG, Harvey C, et al. Screening techniques to identify people at high risk for diabetic foot ulceration. Diabetes Care 2000;23:606–11.
[26] Frykberg RG, Lavery L, Pham H, et al. Role of neuropathy and high foot pressures in diabetic foot ulceration. Diabetes Care 1998;21:1714–9.
[27] Young MJ, Breddy JL, Veves A, Boulton AJM. The prediction of diabetic neuropathic foot ulceration using vibration perception thresholds: a prospective study. Diabetes Care 1994;17: 557–60.
[28] Lavery LA, Armstrong DG, Vela S, et al. Practical criteria for screening patients at high risk for diabetic foot ulceration. Arch Intern Med 1998;158:157–62.
[29] McNeely MJ, Boyko E, Ahroni JH, et al. The independent contributions of diabetic neuropathy and vasculopathy in foot ulceration: how great are the risks? Diabetes Care 1995;18: 216–9.
[30] Kalani M, Brismar K, Fagrell B, et al. Transcutaneous oxygen tension and toe blood pressure as predictors for outcome of diabetic foot ulcers. Diabetes Care 1999;22:147–51.
[31] Pecoraro RE, Ahroni J, Boyko EJ, Stensel VL. Chronology and determinants of tissue repair in diabetic lower-extremity ulcers. Diabetes 1991;40:1305–13.
[32] Boulton AJ, Meneses P, Ennis WJ. Diabetic foot ulcers: a framework for prevention and care. Wound Repair Regen 1999;7:7–17.
[33] Akbari CM, LoGerfo FW. Limb salvage strategies for the high risk foot. Wounds 2000; 12(Suppl B):77B–81B.
[34] Caputo GM, Cavanagh PR, Ulbrecht JS, et al. Assessment and management of foot disease in patients with diabetes. N Engl J Med 1994;331:854–60.
[35] Boulton AJM, Vileikyte L. Pathogenesis of diabetic foot ulceration and measurements of neuropathy. Wounds 2000;12(Suppl B):12B–8B.
[36] Frykberg RG. Biomechanical considerations of the diabetic foot. Lower Extremity 1995;2: 207–14.
[37] Cavanagh PR, Ulbrecht JS, Caputo GM. The biomechanics of the foot in diabetes mellitus. In: Bowker JH, Pfeifer MA, editors. Levin and O'Neal's the diabetic foot. 6th edition. St. Louis (MO): Mosby; 2001. p. 125–96.
[38] Tanenberg RJ, Schumer MP, Greene DA, Pfeifer MA. Neuropathic problems of lower extremities in diabetic patients. In: Bowker JH, Pfeifer MA, editors. Levin and O'Neal's the diabetic foot. 6th edition. St. Louis (MO): Mosby; 2001. p. 33–64.
[39] Cavanagh PR, Ulbrecht JS, Caputo GM. Biomechanical aspects of diabetic foot disease: aetiology, treatment, and prevention. Diabetic Med 1996;13:S17–22.
[40] Pitei DL, Edmonds ME. Foot pressure measurements. Wounds 2000;12(Suppl B):19B–29B.
[41] Ahroni JH, Boyko EJ, Forsberg RC. Clinical correlates of plantar pressure among diabetic veterans. Diabetes Care 1999;22:965–72.
[42] van Schie CHM, Abbott CA, Vileikyte L, et al. A comparative study of the Podotrack, a simple semiquantitative plantar pressure measuring device, and the optical pedobarograph in the assessment of pressures under the diabetic foot. Diabetic Med 1999;16:154–9.
[43] Frykberg RG. Podiatric problems in diabetes. In: Kozak GP, Campbell DR, Frykberg RG, Habershaw GM, editors. Management of diabetic foot problems. 2nd edition. Philadelphia: WB Saunders; 1995. p. 66–87.
[44] Grayson ML, Gibbons GW, Balogh K, et al. Probing to bone in infected pedal ulcers: a clinical sign of underlying osteomyelitis in diabetic patients. JAMA 1995;273:721–3.

[45] Armstrong DG, Lavery LA, Sariaya M, Ashry H. Leukocytosis is a poor indicator of acute osteomyelitis of the foot in diabetes mellitus. J Foot Ankle Surg 1996;35:280–3.
[46] Grayson ML. Diabetic foot infections: antimicrobial therapy. Infect Dis Clin North Am 1995;9: 143–61.
[47] Eneroth M, Apelqvist J, Stenstrom A. Clinical characteristics and outcome in 223 diabetic patients with deep foot infections. Foot Ankle Int 1997;18:716–22.
[48] Lipsky BA. Antibiotic therapy of diabetic foot infections. Wounds 2000;12(Suppl):55B–63B.
[49] Frykberg RG, Veves A. Diabetic foot infections. Diabetes Metab Rev 1996;12:255–70.
[50] Lipsky BA. Osteomyelitis of the foot in diabetic patients. Clin Infect Dis 1997;25:1318–26.
[51] Johnson JE, Kennedy EJ, Shereff MJ, et al. Prospective study of bone, indium-111-labeled white blood cell, and gallium-67 scanning for the evaluation of osteomyelitis in the diabetic foot. Foot Ankle Int 1996;17:10–6.
[52] Blume PA, Dey HM, Daley LJ, et al. Diagnosis of pedal osteomyelitis with Tc-99m HMPAO labeled leukocytes. J Foot Ankle Surg 1997;36:120–6.
[53] Ledermann HP, Morrison WB, Schweitzer ME. Pedal abscesses in patients suspected of having pedal osteomyelitis: analysis with MRI imaging. Radiology 2002;224:649–55.
[54] Unal SN, Birinci H, Baktiroglu S, Cantez S. Comparison of Tc-99m methylene diphosphonate, Tc-99m human immune globulin, and Tc-99m-labeled white blood cell scintigraphy in the diabetic foot. Clin Nucl Med 2001;26:1016–21.
[55] Palestro CJ, Caprioli R, Love C, et al. Rapid diagnosis of pedal osteomyelitis in diabetics with a technetium-99m-labeled monoclonal antigranulocyte antibody. J Foot Ankle Surg 2003;42:2–8.
[56] Eckman MH, Greenfield S, Mackey WC, et al. Foot infections in diabetic patients: decision and cost-effectiveness analyses. JAMA 1995;273:712–20.
[57] Frykberg RG. Diabetic foot ulcerations. In: Frykberg RG, editor. The high risk foot in diabetes mellitus. New York: Churchill Livingstone; 1991. p. 151.
[58] Wagner FW. The dysvascular foot: a system for diagnosis and treatment. Foot Ankle 1981;2:64.
[59] Armstrong DG, Lavery LA, Harkless LB. Validation of a diabetic wound classification system; the contribution of depth, infection, and ischemia to risk of amputation. Diabetes Care 1998;21: 855–9.
[60] Jeffcoate WJ, MacFarlane RM, Fletcher EM. The description and classification of diabetic foot lesions. Diabetic Med 1993;10:676–9.
[61] Oyibo SO, Jude EB, Tarawneh I, et al. A comparison of two diabetic foot ulcer classification systems: the Wagner and the University of Texas wound classification systems. Diabetes Care 2001;24:84–8.
[62] Edmonds ME, Blundell MP, Morris ME, et al. Improved survival of the diabetic foot: the role of a specialised foot clinic. Q J Med 1986;232:763.
[63] Holstein PE, Sorensen S. Limb salvage experience in a multidisciplinary diabetic foot unit. Diabetes Care 1999;22(Suppl 2):B97 103.
[64] Dargis V, Pantelejeva O, Jonushaite A, et al. Benefits of a multidisciplinary approach in the management of recurrent diabetic foot ulceration in Lithuania. Diabetes Care 1999;22:1428–31.
[65] Van Gils CC, Wheeler LA, Mellstrom M, et al. Amputation prevention by vascular surgery and podiatry collaboration in high-risk diabetic and nondiabetic patients: the Operation Desert Foot experience. Diabetes Care 1999;22:678–83.
[66] Pham HT. Wound care in diabetic foot ulceration. Wounds 2000;12(Suppl B):82B–9B.
[67] Steed DL, Donohoe D, Webster MW, Lindsley L. Diabetic Ulcer Study Group: effect of extensive debridement and treatment on the healing of diabetic foot ulcers. J Am Coll Surg 1996;183:61–4.
[68] Alvarez OM, Fernandez-Obregon A, Rogers RS, et al. Chemical debridement of pressure ulcers: a prospective, randomized, comparative trial of collagenase and papain/urea formulations. Wounds 2000;12:15–25.
[69] Falanga V. Wound bed preparation and the role of enzymes: a case for multiple actions of therapeutic agents. Wounds 2002;14:47–57.
[70] Mumcuoglu KY. Clinical applications for maggots in wound care. Am J Clin Dermatol 2001;2: 219–27.

[71] Graninger M, Grassberger M, Galehr E, et al. Biosurgical debridement facilitates healing of chronic skin ulcers. Arch Int Med 2002;162:1906–7.
[72] Hogge J, Krasner D, Nguyen H, et al. The potential benefits of advanced therapeutic modalities in the treatment of diabetic foot wounds. J Am Pod Med Assoc 2000;90:57–65.
[73] Seaman S. Dressing selection in chronic wound management. J Am Pod Med Assoc 2002;92: 24–33.
[74] Donaghue VM, Chrzan JS, Rosenblum BI, et al. Evaluation of a collagen-alginate wound dressing in the management of diabetic foot ulcers. Adv Wound Care 1998;11:114–9.
[75] Hodde J. Naturally occurring scaffolds for soft tissue repair and regeneration. Tissue Eng 2002;8: 295–308.
[76] Brown-Etris M, Cutshall WD, Hiles MC. A new biomaterial derived from small intestine submucosa and developed into a wound matrix device. Wounds 2002;14:150–66.
[77] Steed DL. The role of growth factors in wound healing. Surg Clin North Am 1997;77:575–86.
[78] Wieman TJ, Smiell JM, Su Y. Efficacy and safety of a topical gel formulation of recombinant human platelet-derived growth factor–BB (Becaplermin) in patients with chronic neuropathic diabetic ulcers: a phase III randomized placebo-controlled double-blind study. Diabetes Care 1998;21:822–7.
[79] Hanft JR, Suprenant MS. Healing of chronic foot ulcers in diabetic patients treated with a human fibroblast-derived dermis. J Foot Ankle Surg 2002;41:291–9.
[80] Veves A, Falanga V, Armstrong DG, Sabolinski ML. Graftskin, a human skin equivalent, is effective in the management of noninfected neuropathic diabetic foot ulcers. A prospective randomized multicenter clinical trial. Diabetes Care 2001;24:290–5.
[81] Argenta LC, Morywas MJ. Vacuum-assisted closure: a new method for control and treatment. Clinical experience. Ann Plast Surg 1997;38:563–76.
[82] Clare MP, Fitzgibbons TC, McMullen ST, et al. Experience with vacuum assisted closure negative pressure technique in the treatment of non-healing diabetic and dysvascular wounds. Foot Ankle Int 2002;23:896–901.
[83] Armstrong DG, Lavery LA, Abu-Ramman P, et al. Outcomes of subatmospheric pressure dressing therapy on wounds of the diabetic foot. Ostomy Wound Manage 2002;48:64–8.
[84] Alvarez OM, Rogers RS, Booker JG, Patel M. Effect of noncontact normothermic wound therapy on the healing of neuropathic (diabetic) foot ulcers: an interim analysis of 20 patients. J Foot Ankle Surg 2003;42:30–5.
[85] Karr JC. External thermoregulation of wound associated with lower-extremity osteomyelitis: a pilot study. J Am Podiatric Med Assoc 2003;93:18–22.
[86] Catanzariti AR, Haverstock BD, Grossman JP, Mendocino RW. Off-loading techniques in the treatment of diabetic plantar neuropathic foot ulceration. Adv Wound Care 1999;12:452–8.
[87] Lavery LA, Vela SA, Lavery DC, Quebedeaux TL. Reducing dynamic foot pressures in high-risk diabetic subjects with foot ulcerations. Diabetes Care 1996;19:818–21.
[88] Guzman B, Fisher G, Palladino SJ, Stavosky JW. Pressure-removing strategies in neuropathic ulcer therapy. Clin Pod Med Surg 1994;11:339–53.
[89] Mueller MJ, Diamond JE, Sinacore DR, et al. Total contact casting in treatment of diabetic plantar ulcers. Diabetes Care 1989;12:384.
[90] Shaw JE, Hsi W-L, Ulbrecht JS, et al. Mechanism of plantar unloading in total contact casts: implications, design, and clinical use. Foot Ankle Int 1997;18:809–17.
[91] Armstrong DG, Nguyen HC, Lavery LA, et al. Off-loading the diabetic foot wound: a randomized clinical trial. Diabetes Care 2001;24:1019–22.
[92] Knowles EA, Armstrong DG, Hayat SA, et al. Offloading diabetic foot wounds using the Scotchcast boot: a retrospective study. Ostomy Wound Manage 2002;48:50–3.
[93] Lipsky BA, Berendt AR. Principles and practice of antibiotic therapy of diabetic foot infections. Diabetes Metab Res Rev 2000;16(Suppl 1):S42–6.
[94] Pellizzer G, Strazzabosco M, Presi S, et al. Deep tissue biopsy vs. superficial swab culture monitoring in the microbiological assessment of limb-threatening diabetic foot infection. Diabetic Med 2001;18:822–7.

[95] Lipsky BA, Baker PD, Landon GC, Fernau R. Antibiotic therapy for diabetic foot infections: comparison of two parenteral-to-oral regimens. Clin Infect Dis 1997;24:643–8.
[96] Tan JS, Friedman NM, Hazelton-Miller C, et al. Can aggressive treatment of diabetic foot infections reduce the need for above-ankle amputation? Clin Infect Dis 1996;23:286–91.
[97] Ha Van G, Siney H, Danan J-P, et al. Treatment of osteomyelitis in the diabetic foot:contribution of conservative surgery. Diabetes Care 1996;19:1257–60.
[98] Pomposelli FB, Kansal N, Hamdan AD, et al. A decade of experience with dorsalis pedis artery bypass: analysis of outcome in more than 1000 cases. J Vasc Surg 2003;37:307–15.
[99] Dyet JF, Nicholson AA, Ettles DFE. Vascular imaging and intervention in peripheral arteries in the diabetic patient. Diabetes Metab Res Rev 2000;16(Suppl 1):S16–22.
[100] Faglia E, Favales F, Aldeghi A, et al. Adjunctive systemic hyperbaric oxygen therapy in treatment of severe prevalently ischemic diabetic foot ulcer: a randomized study. Diabetes Care 1996;19: 1338–43.
[101] Kalani M, Jorneskog G, Naderi N, et al. Hyperbaric oxygen (HBO) therapy in treatment of diabetic foot ulcers: long-term follow-up. J Diabetes Complications 2002;16:153–8.
[102] Wang C, Schwaitzberg S, Berliner E, et al. Hyperbaric oxygen for treating wounds: a systematic review of the literature. Arch Surg 2003;138:272–9.
[103] Leslie CA, Sapico FL, Ginunas VJ, Adkins RH. Randomized controlled trial of topical hyperbaric oxygen for treatment of diabetic foot ulcers. Diabetes Care 1988;11:111–5.
[104] Frykberg RG, Giurini J, Habershaw GM, et al. Prophylactic surgery in the diabetic foot. In: Kominsky SJ, editor. Medical and surgical management of the diabetic foot. St. Louis (MO): Mosby Yearbook; 1994. p. 399–439.
[105] Armstrong DG, Frykberg RG. Classifying diabetic foot surgery: toward a rational definition. Diabet Med 2003;20(4):329–31.
[106] Gottrup F, Holstein P, Jorgensen B, et al. A new concept of a multidisciplinary wound healing center and a national expert function of wound healing. Arch Surg 2001;136:765–72.
[107] Frykberg RG, Piaggesi A, Donaghue VM, et al. Difference in treatment of foot ulcerations in Boston, USA, and Pisa, Italy. Diabetes Res Clin Pract 1997;35:21–6.
[108] Giacalone VF, Krych SM, Harkless LB. The University of Texas Health Science Center at San Antonio: experience with foot surgery in diabetics. J Foot Ankle Surg 1994;33:590–7.
[109] Armstrong DG, Lavery LA, Stern S, Harkless LB. Is prophylactic diabetic foot surgery dangerous? J Foot Ankle Surg 1996;35:585–9.
[110] DeNamur C, Pupp G. Diabetic limb salvage: a team approach at a teaching institution. J Am Podiatr Med Assoc 2002;92:457–62.
[111] Blume PA, Paragas LK, Sumpio BE, Attinger CE. Single-stage surgical treatment of noninfected diabetic foot ulcers. Plast Reconstr Surg 2002;109:601–9.
[112] Kumagai SG, Mahoney CR, Fitzgibbons TC, et al. Treatment of diabetic (neuropathic) foot ulcers with two-stage debridement and closure. Foot Ankle Int 1998;19:160–5.
[113] Chaytor ER. Surgical treatment of the diabetic foot. Diabetes Metab Rev 2000;16(Suppl 1): S66–9.
[114] Gill LH. Foot surgery in the patient with diabetes. J South Orthop Assoc 1994;3:261–7.
[115] Catanzariti AR, Blitch EL, Karlock LG. Elective foot and ankle surgery in the diabetic patient. J Foot Ankle Surg 1995;34:23–41.
[116] Baravarian B, Menendez MM, Weinheimer DJ, et al. Subtotal calcanectomy for the treatment of large heel ulceration and calcaneal osteomyelitis in the diabetic patient. J Foot Ankle Surg 1999; 38:194–202.
[117] Armstrong DG, Stackpoole-Shea S, Nguyen H, Harkless LB. Lengthening of the Achilles tendon in diabetic patients who are at high risk for ulceration of the foot. J Bone Joint Surg 1999; 81A:535–8.
[118] Paragas LK, Attinger C, Blume PA. Local flaps. Clin Pod Med Surg 2000;17:267–319.
[119] Bowker JH, San Giovanni TP. Minor and major lower limb amputation in persons with diabetes mellitus. In: Bowker JH, Pfeifer MA, editors. Levin and O'Neal's the diabetic foot. 6th edition. St. Louis (MO): Mosby; 2001. p. 607–35.

[120] Van Damme H, Rorive M, De Noorthout BM, et al. Amputations in diabetic patients: a plea for foot-sparing surgery. Acta Chir Belg 2001;101:123–9.
[121] Connolly JE, Wrobel JS, Anderson RF. Primary closure of infected diabetic foot wounds: a report of closed instillation in 30 cases. J Am Podiatr Med Assoc 2000;90:175–82.
[122] Armstrong DG, Findlow AH, Oyibo SO, Boulton AJM. The use of absorbable antibiotic-impregnated calcium sulphate pellets in the management of diabetic foot infections. Diabet Med 2001;18:942–3.
[123] Schessel ES, Lombardi CM, Dennis LN. External constant tension expansion of soft tissue for the treatment of ulceration of the foot and ankle. J Foot Ankle Surg 2000;39:321–8.
[124] American Diabetes Association. Preventive foot care in people with diabetes. Diabetes Care 2002;25(Suppl 1):S69–70.
[125] Uccioli L, Faglia E, Monticone G, et al. Manufactured shoes in the prevention of diabetic foot ulcers. Diabetes Care 1995;18:1376–8.
[126] Praet SFE, Louwerens J-WK. The influence of shoe design on plantar pressures in neuropathic feet. Diabetes Care 2003;26:441–5.
[127] Reiber GE, Smith DG, Wallace C, et al. Effect of therapeutic footwear on foot reulceration in patients with diabetes: a randomized controlled trial. JAMA 2002;287:2552–8.
[128] Cavanagh PR, Boulton AJ, Sheehan P, et al. Therapeutic footwear in patients with diabetes [letter]. JAMA 2002;288:1231.

CLINICS IN PODIATRIC MEDICINE AND SURGERY

Clin Podiatr Med Surg
20 (2003) 729–740

Imaging modalities of the diabetic foot

Enzo J. Sella[a,*], Dawn M. Grosser[b]

[a]*Connecticut Orthopaedic Specialists, 2408 Whitney Avenue, Hamden, CT 06518, USA*
[b]*Department of Orthopaedics and Rehabilitation, Yale University, 800 Howard Avenue, New Haven, CT 06520, USA*

Diabetic foot disease can be organized into three primary categories based on pathogenesis: neuropathic, infectious, and vascular. The cost of these various pathologic processes to the patient cannot be underestimated (ie, diabetic foot conditions are the cause of more hospitalization than any other aspect of the disease, with a mean stay of 6 weeks) [1–3]. At least 6% of these patients will eventually need amputation, making early, accurate diagnosis crucial [4]. In this article, imaging as it relates to diagnosing the neuropathic and infectious aspects of diabetic foot disease will be described.

Diabetic osteoarthropathy causes painless, destructive changes and deformities in joints with underlying neurologic deficits. The most common medical condition associated with the development of a Charcot joint is diabetes mellitus, with approximately 5% of patients who have diabetes developing this in their lifetime [5]. The neuropathy can be sensory, motor, or autonomic. It involves the nervous, vascular, and musculoskeletal systems and it affects the patient's perception of pain and ability to respond appropriately. There is loss of myelinated and unmyelinated nerve fibers secondary to accumulation of sorbitol (a breakdown product of glucose) in the nerve tissue and ischemia to peripheral nerves as a result of occlusive disease in the vasa nervorum. Both processes lead to impaired sensation, pain, temperature, and proprioception [6]. Autonomic denervation leads to a loss of vasoconstrictor control, which along with arterial calcification and thickening of the basement membrane causes increased blood volume and increased transit time in the foot. Blood flow has been shown to be five times greater in the neuropathic compared with the nonneuropathic foot [7]. The high rate of flow produces A-V shunting with subsequent bone demineralization and breakdown. Joint degeneration and subluxations cause a natural hyperemic response promoting softening and resorption of debris and normal bone. Further trauma to an osteoporotic, insensate foot produces more destruc-

* Corresponding author.
E-mail address: enzojsella@hotmail.com (E.J. Sella).

doi:10.1016/S0891-8422(03)00070-3

tion, creating a vicious cycle of breakdown and attempted repair. This process occurs more frequently at points of the greatest stress. The midfoot is affected 60% of the time, followed by the metatarsophalangeal joints, 30%, and tibiotalar joint, 10% [8]. Besides diabetes, other causes of neuropathic arthropathy include spinal cord injuries, paraplegia, multiple sclerosis, syringomyelia, intraarticular injection of steroids, congenital insensitivity to pain, tertiary syphilis, alcoholism, and leprosy [9].

At the onset of diabetic osteoarthropathy, the clinical appearance is one of warmth, swelling, and erythema, which may be clinically indistinguishable from osteomyelitis; however, both conditions may occur simultaneously. The differential diagnosis includes neuropathic osteoarthropathy, arthritis, gout, and pes planus. Ninety-five percent of patients with osteomyelitis have an associated ulcer, making the clinical diagnosis of osteomyelitis in a patient without an ulcer unlikely [4]. The clinical diagnosis of osteomyelitis in the diabetic foot is 100% specific when an ulcer probes to bone, but is otherwise insensitive, with failure to detect osteomyelitis 68% of the time. Laboratory tests are no more accurate than clinical judgment [10]. It is important therefore to confirm or disprove the diagnosis of diabetic osteoarthropathy versus osteomyelitis by the judicious use of appropriate imaging studies, such as plain films, diphosphonate scans, WBC-labeled scintigraphy, bone marrow scans, computerized tomography, and magnetic resonance imaging.

Plain radiographs

Plain radiographs should be the initial screening exam for any patient suspected of osteoarthropathy or osteomyelitis even though it is the least sensitive of all imaging modalities (Fig. 1) [2]. Radiographic findings may be used to make the diagnosis of a Charcot joint and to stage the progression [11]. Stage 0 is a clinical stage manifested by localized heat, swelling, redness, and increased perfusion. Stage 1 shows localized osteoporosis, subchondral cysts, erosions, and diastasis.

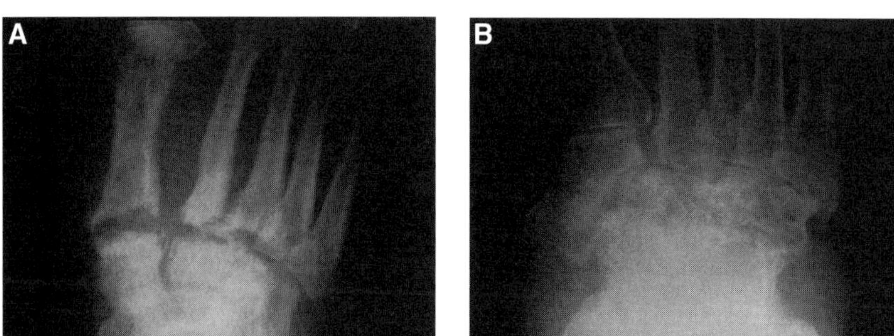

Fig. 1. (*A*) Osteomyelitis with intramedullary spread into the first metatarsal. (*B*) Charcot osteoarthropathy with cystic changes and erosions.

Table 1
Clinical and radiographic staging of Charcot

Stages	Findings
0	Clinical: warmth, swelling, rythema, perfusion
1	Radiographic: osteopenia, cysts, erosions, diastasis
2	Joint subluxations
3	Joint dislocations
4	Consolidation and fusion

Adapted from Sella EJ, Barette C. Staging of neuroarthropathy along the median column of the foot in the diabetic patient. J Foot Ankle Surg 1999;38(1):34–40.

Stage 2 reveals further progression to subluxation and stage 3 results in dislocation. In stage 4, evidence of sclerosis and fusion is present (Table 1, Figs. 2–5).

Radiographic signs of osteoarthropathy and osteomyelitis are often interchangeable, particularly when the atrophic form of osteoarthropathy is present [2]. These signs consist of demineralization, periosteal reaction, and bony destruction (Fig. 1). The same findings are also seen in fractures, joint deformities, and tumors. Fig. 1 emphasizes the difficulty in distinguishing between osteoarthropathy and osteomyelitis. Both films show midfoot erosions and articular and periarticular breakdown; however; in Fig. 1A there is intramedullary involvement of the first metatarsal indicative of hematogenous osteomyelitis. When it occurs in the diabetic foot, osteomyelitis affects adjacent joints and does not become intramedullary. Fig. 1B is an example of stage 2 Charcot without osteomyelitis. Some 30% to 50% of bone must be destroyed before osteomyelitis can be diagnosed radiographically [3]. It is therefore important to maintain a high index of suspicion to make the proper diagnosis in the early stages of the disease

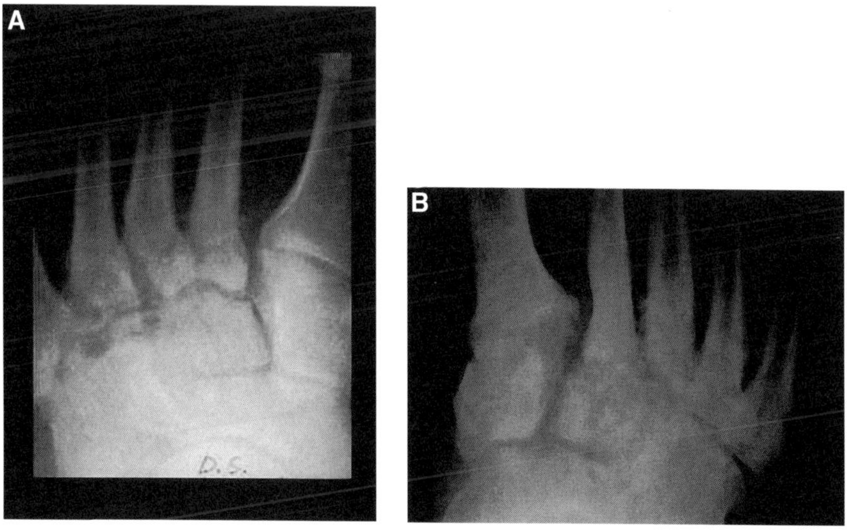

Fig. 2. (*A,B*) Stage 1: Charcot osteoarthropathy. Erosions, cystic changes without subluxations.

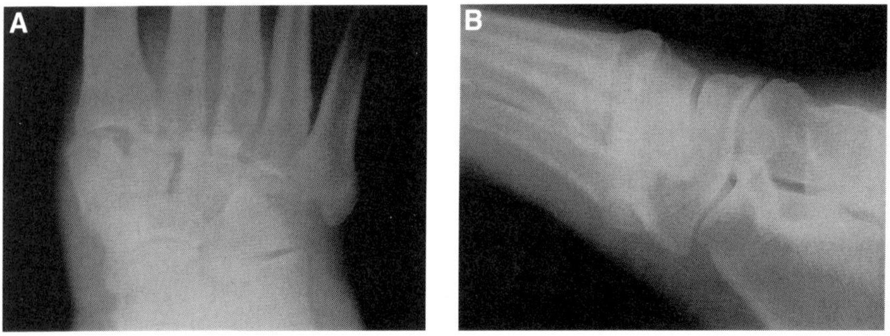

Fig. 3. (*A,B*) Stage 2: Subluxations first and second cuneiform-metatarsal joints.

process, because if the diagnosis is made early, 25% of patients may not develop deformity [11].

Plain radiographs used to diagnose osteomyelitis in patients with foot ulcers have a sensitivity of 28% to 93%, and a specificity of 25% to 92% (Table 2) [2,12]. The differentiation between osteoarthropathy and osteomyelitis cannot be made consistently, and other imaging modalities are needed for clarification.

Diphosphonate scanning

The bone scan is more sensitive than plain radiography, but not specific for diagnosing osteomyelitis. The three-phase bone scan is made up of an initial postinjection radionuclide angiogram, then a "blood-pool" image, followed by a delayed static image 2 to 3 hours or 5 to 7 hours later [20].

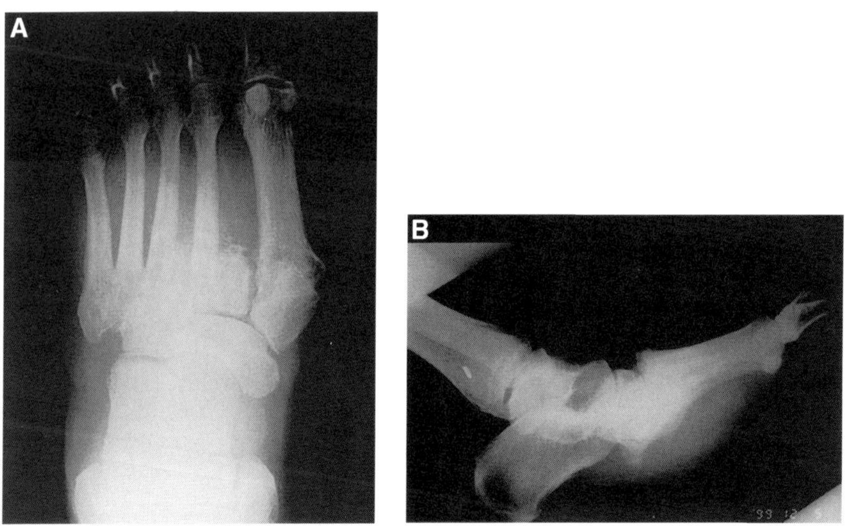

Fig. 4. (*A,B*) Stage 3: Dislocations cuneiform-metatarsal joints. Early rocker-bottom.

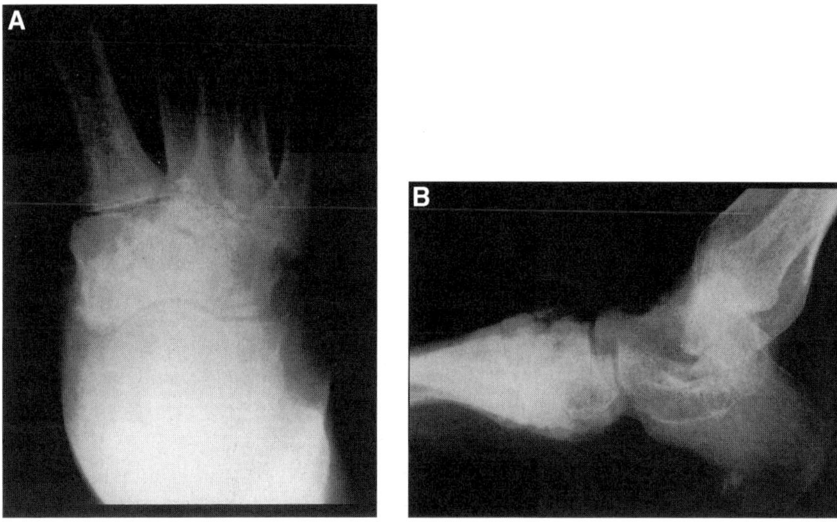

Fig. 5. (*A,B*) Stage 4: Fusion of midfoot.

The image produced by bone scan is affected by rate of bone turnover, capillary permeability, tissue perfusion, and regional blood flow. Conditions producing hyperemia or ischemia will affect the bone scan. For example, in osteoarthropathy, fractures, and long-standing soft tissue infections, which are often hyperemic, there is a high false-positive rate. Therefore, although a positive bone scan is not necessarily indicative of osteomyelitis, a negative study excludes it with a higher degree of probability [3]. However, there are still some studies that shed doubt on the predictability of a negative bone scan. One prospective study by Shults et al [5] reported on a three-phase scan in 25 patients with biopsy proven osteomyelitis and found a low specificity, 43%. Newman also found, in a similar study, a specificity of only 39% [10]. None of the patients in these two studies had any evidence of systemic osteomyelitis.

Table 2
Osteomyelitis by radiography

Study (plain radiographs)	*N*	Sensitivity (%)	Specificity (%)
Park et al [13]	39	62	69
Seldin et al [14]	30	93	50
Larcos et al [15]	49	43	83
Newman et al [10]	35	28	92
Yuh et al [16]	24	72	60
Kennan et al [17]	77	69	82
Wang et al [18]	50	52	69
Caprioli et al [19]	14	90	25
Shults et al [5]	32	52	67

Adapted from Gold RH, Tong Dominic JF, Crim JR, Seeger L. Imaging the diabetic foot. Skeletal Radiol 1995;24:563–71.

When osteoarthropathy is present, the midfoot and tibiotalar joints usually demonstrate more bony destruction and less anatomic resolution. The scintigraphic abnormalities precede and are often more extensive than the radiographic changes [21]. (Table 3 demonstrates the high sensitivity but low specificity of bone scans found by various authors.) The three-phase bone scan is usually positive regardless of whether osteomyelitis is present. To improve the specificity of bone scans in the midfoot, some studies have evaluated the use of additional methods, such as computerized analysis of the bone scan (ie, dynamic bone imaging and dual tracer). Dynamic bone imaging or computerized blood flow studies (CBFS), similar to three-phase bone scan, involves injection of diphosphonate. Data is then acquired at one frame per second for the first 60 seconds and then one frame per minute for 24 minutes. This data is quantified according to "time-activity curves" for the various regions of interest during three phases: arterial (phase I), blood-pool (phase II), and bone uptake (phase III), which occur during the 1 to 25 minutes after injection. Ratios are calculated for each region of interest (ROI), which is proportional to the amount of blood flow to the various regions. This number is then compared with a standard of normal values to determine increased blood flow. This additional method enhances the specificity of the bone scan because in cases of acute osteomyelitis there is intense hyperemia in all three phases of the involved area as well as in the region of interest proximal to the infected area (ie, distal tibia). In uninfected Charcot joints, the hyperemic phases were identical to those of osteomyelitis in the involved areas, except in the distal tibia where hyperemic changes were limited to the first and second phases, whereas the third phase demonstrated normal flow, thereby affording a method to distinguish between the two conditions [1,24].

Other agents that are known to localize in areas of infection, such as gallium and labeled leukocytes, have been explored through dual tracer studies in an attempt to enhance specificity. Unfortunately, results in the neuropathic foot have been disappointing [25]. Gallium-67 citrate was found to accumulate in areas of increased bone turnover but demonstrated similar sensitivity and specificity as the

Table 3
Osteomyelitis by three-phase bone scan

Study (^{99}Tc-MDP *bone scan*)	*N*	Sensitivity (%)	Specificity (%)
Park et al [13]	36	83	75
Seldin et al [14]	30	94	79
Larcos et al [15]	49	93	43
Maurer et al [22]	13	75	56
Yuh et al [16]	24	94	18
Kennan et al [17]	77	100	38
Newman et al [10]	35	69	39
Weinstein et al [23]	32	69	83
Caprioli et al [19]	10	100	25
Shults et al [5]	25	67	43

Adapted from Gold RH, Tong Dominic JF, Crim JR, Seeger L. Imaging the diabetic foot. Skeletal Radiol 1995;24:563–71.

Table 4
Three-phase versus four-phase bone scan

$N = 21$	Sensitivity	Specificity	Accuracy
Three-phase	100%	73%	80%
Four-phase	80%	87%	85%

Adapted from Alazraki N, Dries D, Datz F, Lawrence P, Greenberg E, Taylor Jr A. Value of 24 hour image (four phase bone scan) in assessing osteomyelitis in patients with peripheral vascular disease. J Nucl Med 1985;26:711–7.

three-phase bone scan when evaluating infection in Charcot joints and is therefore not a reliable agent to confirm the diagnosis of osteomyelitis in diabetic osteoarthropathy [25,26].

The four-phase bone scan adds an additional static image at 24 hours. In normal bone, tracer accumulation finishes within 3 to 4 hours after injection, but in immature, woven bone, as in osteomyelitis, uptake continues for several hours, which would be missed in the three-phase scan. If osteomyelitis is present, the 24-hour images should show an increased lesion-to-background-activity ratio compared with earlier images [2]. However, the problem arises that immature woven bone is not limited to infection but also found in fractures and in other types of bone remodeling, such as Charcot osteoarthropathy. In the study by Alazraki [20], there was no significant improvement in results using the four-phase bone scan (Table 4). Given the routinely low specificity and negative predictive value of bone scans, and the minor difference in three-phase versus four-phase bone scans, additional studies are indicated in patients suspected of having osteomyelitis.

Leukocyte-labeled studies

Multiple studies have shown that leukocyte scans generally have higher sensitivity and specificity than bone scans or radiographs (Table 5).

One drawback is that leukocytes accumulate in the uninfected Charcot joint [26]. This is initially the result of an early inflammatory response to micro-

Table 5
Osteomyelitis detected by leukocyte scan

Study(^{111}In white blood cell scan)	N	Sensitivity (%)	Specificity (%)
Larcos et al [15]	51	79	78
Schauwecker et al [27]	35	100	83
Maurer et al [22]	13	75	89
Keenan et al [17]	46	100	78
Seabold et al [25]	14	80	54
Newman et al [10]	35	89	69

Adapted from Gold RH, Tong Dominic JF, Crim JR, Seeger L. Imaging the diabetic foot. Skeletal Radiol 1995;24:563–71.

Table 6
Plain radiographs, three-phase scan, HMPAO

	Sensitivity (%)	Specificity (%)
Plain radiographs	55	57
Three-phase bone scan	75	29
HMPAO WBC scan	90	80

fractures with polymorphonuclear cells. But in a chronic Charcot joint, the synovial effusion is mononuclear, therefore the polymorphonuclear uptake is more likely secondary to the hematopoietically active marrow that is normally involved in the repair process [24,28,29].

There is also a difference in sensitivity and specificity depending on the location of the pathology. Forefoot scans are more easily interpreted because of better spatial resolution as the bony anatomy is much better outlined than in the midfoot where there is bony overlap. Where there is no clear anatomic definition, it is difficult to differentiate soft tissue from bone infection using leukocyte scans. In an attempt to overcome this difficulty, Larcos et al [15] used the combination of methylene diphosphonate (MDP) and labeled leukocytes and classified the results as positive for osteomyelitis when the leukocyte uptake was of "proportionately greater intensity" than the diphosphonate bone scan However, in spite of using this differential uptake criterion between ^{99}Tc-MDP and ^{111}In-WBC, the combined interpretation did not significantly improve the sensitivity or specificity of the study: 89% and 50% respectively. Although there may not be significant advantage in the acute setting for combined interpretation using the three-phase bone scan and labeled leukocyte scan, a study by Newman [10] shows promising results in following the progress of antibiotic therapy. In this study, the scans were repeated during the course of treatment and the bone scan remained positive; the labeled leukocyte scan reverted to normal as early as 2 weeks. The combined interpretation of these studies is a good technique to monitor the response to therapy.

Besides the poor spatial resolution of the leukocyte scans, another disadvantage is that it takes 2 days to complete. It is possible to label WBCs with 99mTc using the carrier hexamethyl-propylene-amine-oxime (HMPAO). This provides improved spatial resolution and the ability to perform labeling and imaging on the same day, usually within 4 hours [30,31]. Blume et al [32] prospectively evaluated the usefulness of 99m-HMPAO-labeled leukocytes for the diagnosis of pedal osteomyelitis in comparison with plain films and the three-phase bone scan. There was improved sensitivity and specificity with HMPAO (Table 6).

Table 7
WBC scan versus sulfur colloid scan

	WBC scan	Sulfur colloid scan
Infected Charcot	+	–
Uninfected Charcot	+	+

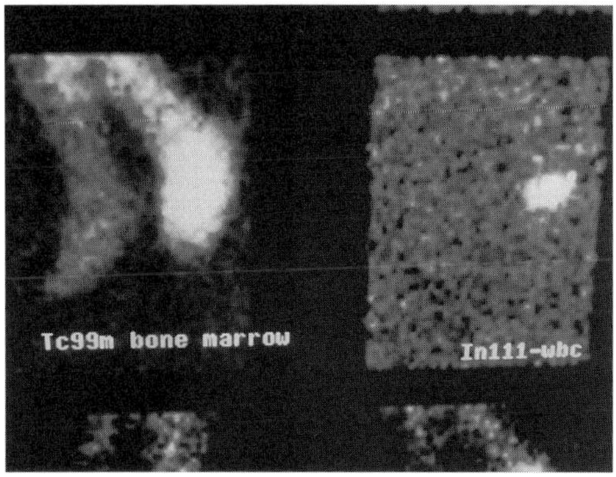

Fig. 6. Increased uptake of bone marrow scan and Indium-111 scan. Negative for osteomyelitis.

Moreover, they found that HMPAO labeled leukocyte scan accurately detected acute and chronic osteomyelitis in patients with diabetic neuropathy and vascular insufficiency, and neither intravenous nor oral antibiotics adversely affected the sensitivity [32]

Other combined studies have been evaluated in an attempt to improve the specificity of leukocyte scans. For example, interpreting labeled leukocyte imaging along with sulfur colloid marrow images has been shown to enhance the specificity and reduce the number of false positives. Infection suppresses normal bone marrow activity but increases leukocyte uptake. Therefore, in the presence of infection the leukocyte scan will be positive but the sulfur colloid marrow scan will be negative with a subsequent disconcordant result (Table 7) [33,34].

Leukocyte combined with marrow imaging is superior to leukocyte and bone imaging alone or in combination for the purpose of distinguishing between osteomyelitis and Charcot osteoarthropathy (Fig. 6) [28]. One study found the sensitivity, specificity, and accuracy to be as high as 95%, 93%, and 94% respectively [35].

Computerized tomography

Before the use of MR imaging, CT scan was useful for detecting early bony erosion and the extent of infection in the bone and soft tissue most clearly in the plantar aspect of the foot. It allowed localization for the most appropriate site for debridement or amputation [2]. CT may show sequestra, cortical destruction, periosteal new bone formation, and small foci of gas within bone better than MRI, but it cannot distinguish between pus, granulation tissue, inflammation, or fibrosis [4]. However, there has been no large study done comparing the two for the evaluation of osteomyelitis. Berquist et al [36] found that MR imaging demonstrates the extent of infection more definitively than CT, which may be helpful in

Table 8
WBC scan versus MR imaging

	Sensitivity (%)	Specificity (%)
Labeled white cell scan	100	67
MR imaging	29	78

the preoperative evaluation. Therefore, there is currently no indication to use CT rather than MR imaging for diagnosing osteomyelitis in the diabetic foot.

Magnetic resonance imaging

Magnetic resonance imaging is affected by the stage and degree of activity of the Charcot osteoarthropathy process. One study reported that MR imaging accurately excluded osteomyelitis superimposed on the neuropathic joint with 100% specificity [37]. Seabold et al [25] stated, however, that Charcot and osteomyelitis are indistinguishable by MR imaging. MR imaging appears to provide good sensitivity but questionable specificity (ie, a negative study excludes osteomyelitis with a high degree of certainty but a positive study is not diagnostic). MR imaging is best used to determine the extent of osteomyelitis and to plan surgery after the diagnosis has already been made. Also, an MR image is more useful for the evaluation of the forefoot, whereas bone marrow scan/leukocyte imaging is better in the midfoot and hindfoot [38].

Labeled WBC scintigraphy is superior to MR imaging for the diagnosis of clinically unsuspected osteomyelitis in the patient who has diabetes, and a negative white cell scan provides strong evidence against infection (Table 8) [10]. But as discussed earlier, a positive study needs to be followed by a sulfur colloid scan to confirm the diagnosis of infection.

Summary

Charcot osteoarthropathy is a devastating process that occurs in the diabetic foot. It must be distinguished from other conditions, such as osteomyelitis, with efficiency and accuracy. The prognosis and treatment depends on it. Charcot progresses along four radiographically identifiable stages; therefore, plain films should be the first step in the evaluation. When osteomyelitis is suspected, a three-phase bone scan may allow clear enough anatomic detail to diagnosis bony involvement compared with soft tissue in the forefoot. In the midfoot, a three-phase bone scan alone is not specific enough to distinguish between Charcot and osteomyelitis. Enhancing the bone scans by adding an additional phase (four-phase) or tracer (gallium) does not appear to improve specificity significantly. Computerized bone flow studies may be more helpful in making the distinction, particularly in acute presentation. A CT scan is not indicated because the MR image will better define the anatomic extent of the process for preoperative planning. The combined WBC scans and sulfur colloid marrow scans show improved specificity and can distinguish between Charcot and osteomyelitis. Combined leukocyte scan with bone marrow imaging is superior to leukocyte and bone scan alone or in combination for detecting infection in the neuropathic foot. The combined leukocyte scan and bone marrow imaging is the current gold standard for evaluating the presence of diabetic foot infection versus osteo-arthropathy, and MR imagine is the anatomic gold standard that may be used to define the extent of the process.

References

[1] Gandsman EJ, Deutsch SD, Kahn CB, et al. Differentiation of Charcot joint from osteomyelitis through dynamic bone imaging. Nucl Med Commun 1990;11:45–53.
[2] Gold RH, Tong Dominic JF, Crim JR, Seeger L. Imaging the diabetic foot. Skeletal Radiol 1995; 24:563–71.
[3] Palestro CJ, Tomas MB. In: Freeman LM, editor. Scientific evaluation of the diabetic foot. Nuclear medicine annual. Philadelphia: Lippincott Williams & Wilkins; 2000. p. 143–72.
[4] Boutin RD, Brossman J, Sartoris DJ, et al. Update on imaging of orthopedic infections. Orthop Clin North Am 1998;29(1):41–66.
[5] Shults DW, Hunter GC, McIntyre KE, et al. Value of radiographs and bone scans in determining the need for therapy in diabetic patients with foot ulcers. Am J Surg 1989;158:525–30.
[6] Horowitz SH. Diabetic neuropathy. Clin Orthop 1993;296:78–85.
[7] Archer AG, Roberts VC, Watkins PJ. Blood flow patterns in painful diabetic neuropathy. Diabetologia 1984;27(6):563–7.
[8] Brodsky JW. The diabetic foot. In: Coughlin MJ, Mann RA, editors. 6th edition. Surgery of the Foot and Ankle, Vol. 2. St. Louis (MO): Mosby; 1999. p. 877–955.
[9] Frykberg RG, Hozack GP. Neuropathic arthropathy in the diabetic foot. Am Fam Physician 1978;May:105–13.
[10] Newman LG, Waller J, Palestro CJ, et al. Leukocyte scanning with IN-111 is superior to magnetic resonance imaging in diagnosis of clinically unsuspected osteomyelitis in diabetic foot ulcers. Diabetes Care 1992;15:1527–30.
[11] Sella EJ, Barette C. Staging of neuroarthropathy along the median column of the foot in the diabetic patient. J Foot Ankle Surg 1999;38(1):34–40.
[12] Newman LG. Imaging techniques in the diabetic foot. Clin Podiatr Med Surg 1995;12:75–86.
[13] Park HM, Wheat J, Siddiqui AR, et al. Scintigraphic evaluation of diabetic osteomyelitis. J Nucl Med 1982;23:569–73.
[14] Seldin DW, Heiken JP, Feldman F, et al. Effect of soft-tissue pathology on detection of pedal osteomyelitis in diabetics. J Nucl Med 1985;26:988–93.
[15] Larcos G, Brown ML, Sutton RT. Diagnosis of osteomyelitis of the foot in diabetic patients: value of 111-leukocyte scintigraphy. AJR Am J Roentgenol 1991;157:527–31.
[16] Yuh WTC, Corson JD, Baraniewski HM, et al. Osteomyelitis of the foot in diabetic patients: evaluation with plain film, ^{99m}Tc-MDP bone scintigraphy and MR imaging. AJR Am J Roentgenol 1989;152:795–800.
[17] Kennan AM, Tindel NL, Alavi A. Diagnosis of pedal osteomyelitis in diabetic patients using current scintigraphic techniques. Arch Intern Med 1989;149:2262–6.
[18] Wang A, Weinstein D, Greenfield L, et al. MRI and diabetic foot infections. Magn Reson Imaging 1990;3:219–30.
[19] Caprioli R, Cournoyer RW, Testa J, et al. Prompt diagnosis of suspected osteomyelitis by utilizing percutaneous bone culture. J Foot Surg 1986;25:263–9.
[20] Alazraki N, Dries D, Datz F, et al. Value of a 24-hour image (four-phase bone scan) in assessing osteomyelitis in patients with peripheral vascular disease. J Nucl Med 1985;26:711–7.

[21] Eymontt MJ, Alavi A, Dalinka MK, et al. Bone scintigraphy in diabetic osteoarthropathy. Radiology 1981;140:475–7.
[22] Maurer AH, Millmond SH, Knight LC, et al. Infection in diabetic osteoarthropathy: use of indium-labeled leukocytes for diagnosis. Radiology 1986;161:221–5.
[23] Weinstein D, Wang A, Chambers R, et al. Evaluation of magnetic resonance imaging in the diagnosis of osteomyelitis in diabetic foot infections. Foot Ankle 1993;14:18–22.
[24] Knight D, Gray HW, McKillop JH, et al. Imaging for infection: caution required with the Charcot joint. Eur J Nucl Med 1988;13:523–6.
[25] Seabold JE, Flickinger FW, Simon CS. Indium-111-leukocyte/technetium-99m-MDP bone and magnetic resonance imaging: difficulty of diagnosing osteomyelitis in patients with neuropathic osteoarthropathy. J Nucl Med 1990;31:549–56.
[26] Schauwecker DS, Park HM, Mock BH, et al. Evaluation of complicating osteomyelitis with Tc-99m MDP, In-111 granulocytes, and Ga-67 citrate. J Nucl Med 1984;25(8):849–53.
[27] Schauwecker DS, Park HM, Burt RW, et al. Combined bone scintigraphy and indium-111 leukocyte scans in neuropathic foot disease. J Nucl Med 1988;29:1651–5.
[28] Palestro CJ, Mehta HH, Patel M, et al. Marrow versus infection in the Charcot joint: Indium-111 leukocyte and technetium-99m sulfur colloid scintigraphy. J Nucl Med 1998;39(2):346–50.
[29] Tomas MB, Patel M, Marwin SE, et al. The diabetic foot. Br J Radiol 2000;April:443–50.
[30] Devillers A, Moissan A, Hennion F, et al. Contribution of technetium-99m hexamethylpropylene amine oxime labeled leukocyte scintigraphy to the diagnosis of diabetic foot infection. Eur J Nucl Med 1998;25(2):132–8.
[31] Fox IM, Zeiger L. Tc-99m-HMPAO leukocyte scintigraphy for the diagnosis of osteomyelitis in diabetic foot infections. J Foot Ankle Surg 1993;32(6):591–4.
[32] Blume PA, Dey HM, Daley LJ, et al. Diagnosis of pedal osteomyelitis with Tc-99 HMPAO labeled leukocytes. J Foot Ankle Surg 1997;36:120–6.
[33] Palestro CJ, Torres MA. Radionuclide imaging in orthopedic infections. Semin Nucl Med 1997;27(4):334–45.
[34] King AD, Peters AM, Stuttle AWJ, et al. Imaging of bone infection with labeled white blood cells: role of contemporaneous bone marrow imaging. Eur J Nucl Med 1990;17:148–51.
[35] Achong DM, Oates E. The computer-generated bone marrow subtraction image: a valuable adjunct to combined In-111 WBC/Tc99m in sulfur colloid scintigraphy for musculoskeletal infection. Clin Nucl Med 1994;19(3):188–93.
[36] Berquist TH, Brown ML, Fitzgerald RH, et al. Magnetic resonance imaging: application in musculoskeletal infection. Magn Reson Imaging 1985;3:219–30.
[37] Beltram J, Campanini S, Knight C, et al. The diabetic foot: magnetic resonance imaging evaluation. Skeletal Radiol 1990;19:37–41.
[38] Lipman BT, Collier BD, Carrera GF, et al. Detection of osteomyelitis in the neuropathic foot: nuclear medicine, MRI, and conventional radiology. Clin Nucl Med 1998;23:77–82.

CLINICS IN PODIATRIC MEDICINE AND SURGERY

Clin Podiatr Med Surg 20 (2003) 741–756

External fixation in the management of Charcot neuroarthropathy

Gary Peter Jolly, DPM[a], Thomas Zgonis, DPM[a,*], Vasilios Polyzois, MD[b]

[a]The Center for Reconstructive Foot Surgery, 440 New Britain Avenue, Plainville, CT 06062, USA
[b]Thriassion General Hospital, Elefsina, Greece

Charcot neuroarthropathy is a destructive process involving the foot and ankle in which microfractures and soft tissue disruption occur. If unprotected, a breakdown in the structural integrity of the foot and ankle is likely to occur. This phenomenon was first described by Musgrave in 1703 and was attributed to venereal disease [1]. Jean Martin Charcot identified the disease in neuropathic patients with tertiary syphilis but it was not until 1936 when the disease was recognized in the diabetic population [2,3]. Charcot neuroarthropathy presents only in the presence of sensory neuropathy. It will affect approximately 13% of all diabetic neuropathic patients. It may also present in those patients who have neuropathy of other etiologies. However, in those patients with disorders, such as spinal dysraphism, which preclude ambulation, neuroarthropathy is rarely seen [4–7].

Several theories have been advanced over the past two centuries regarding the etiology of Charcot neuroarthropathy. These include Virchow's theory (German), which attributes the breakdown in the foot to trauma and Charcot's (French) theory, which proposes that insensitivity and the loss of proprioception is primarily responsible for its development. Current thinking suggests that an autonomic neuropathy, which develops in concert with the sensory loss, produces a cutaneous-osseous shunting. This hyperemic interosseous state within the tarsal bones results in a reduction of bone stiffness and reduced bone mineral density, and predisposes individuals with neuropathy to pathological fracture. As seductive as this theory is, it cannot completely explain the phenomenon of acute Charcot neuroarthropathy, because in some individuals there are dislocations that occur without significant concomitant fracture (Fig. 1). Associated with diabetes mellitus are well known changes in the cross-linking of connective tissue, associated with glycosylation, which has been shown to reduce the elasticity of tendons and skin. It may

* Corresponding author.
E-mail address: thomaszgonis@yahoo.com (T. Zgonis).

0891-8422/03/$ – see front matter
doi:10.1016/S0891-8422(03)00071-5

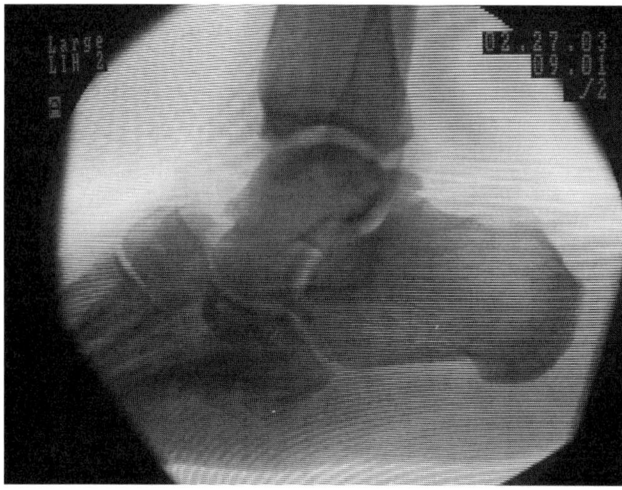

Fig. 1. A radiograph of an acute Charcot dislocation of the midfoot without significant fracture.

be postulated that glycosylation may also affect the tensile strength of ligaments, thereby increasing the risk of dislocation of the midfoot and hindfoot [8–13].

Regardless of the etiology, breakdown of the foot occurs swiftly in the presence of sustained weight-bearing. The forces acting on the foot include the patient's own body weight driving through the tibia, the pull of the triceps, which causes the rearfoot to plantarflex at the level of the breakdown, and the reactive ground forces that drive the forefoot upwards, all contributing to the deformation of the tarsus (Fig. 2).

Although most patients who develop Charcot neuroarthropathy experience their fractures and dislocations insidiously, there is a subset of individuals who

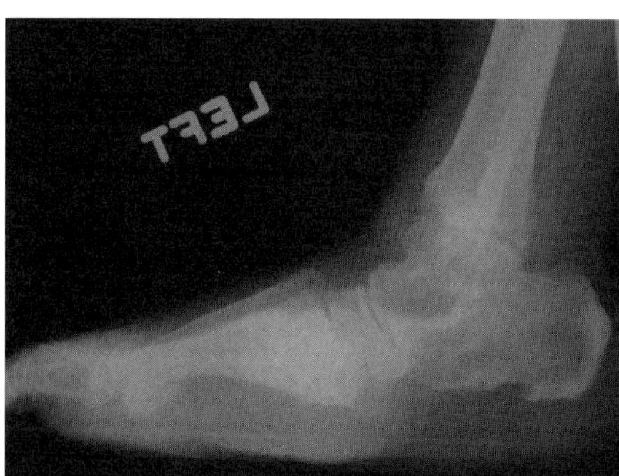

Fig. 2. A lateral radiograph showing a midfoot breakdown. Note the plantarflexing effect of the pull of the triceps on position of the talus and calcaneus.

experience acute traumatic episodes, resulting in ankle fractures, calcaneal fractures, and other more complex injury patterns. The rules of fracture management do not always apply in patients who have diabetic sensory neuropathy and reduced bone mineral densities. Lag screws and plates should be used judiciously in these cases because thread purchase is difficult in soft bone and failure of internal fixation in these settings is high (Fig. 3). In cases where there is minimal displacement and the fractures are stable, the use of a well-padded cast and a course of strict non–weight-bearing may be sufficient to permit healing. The use of forceful closed reductions should be avoided because pressures applied to the foot and leg may lead to soft tissue injury and eventual necrosis. Open reduction and internal or external fixation would be preferable to a forced closed reduction.

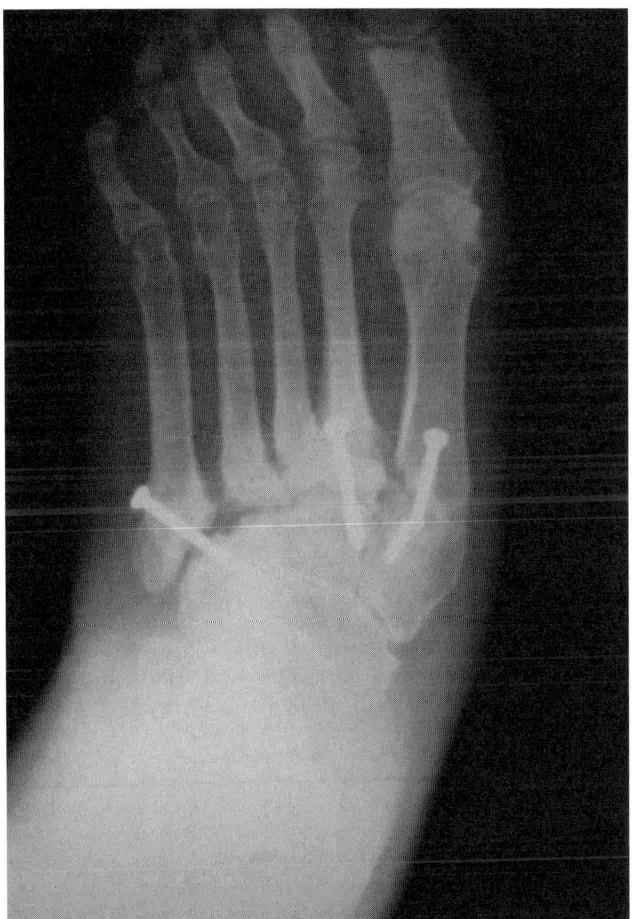

Fig. 3. Radiographs showing complete failure of internal fixation in maintaining reduction of a Lisfranc dislocation associated with Charcot neuroarthropathy.

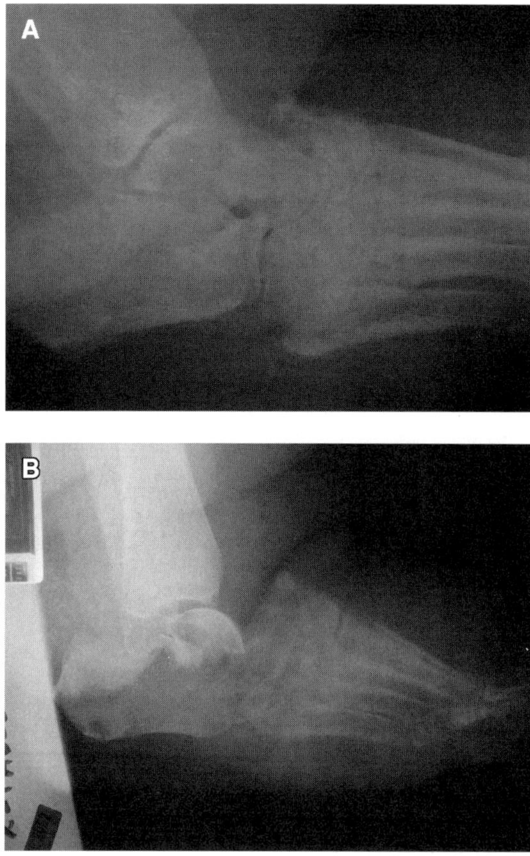

Fig. 4. (*A*) A lateral radiograph showing an old Charcot event affecting the lesser tarsus. (*B*) A radiograph of the same 5 years later demonstrating a second acute event with dissolution of the talus and navicular.

It has been suggested that once an acute Charcot event consolidates, the foot is safe from reinjury. Though this may be true for most patients, exceptions do occur (Fig. 4). A question that begs is whether an acute Charcot event and consolidation changes the physical properties of the bones involved in the injury by increasing cortical stiffness and bone mineral densities.

Clinical stages of Charcot neuroarthropathy

Eichenholz, in 1966, was the first to describe a staging system for Charcot neuroarthropathy [14]. The foot was thought to pass through three distinct clinical stages during the course of a Charcot event. Stage I has been called the acute phase and includes the development of hyperemia and osteopenia with resultant microfracture and early diastasis. During the first stage, patients may complain of vague foot pain or the event may be completely painless. The foot becomes edematous and warm, and radiographs taken during this period may reveal subtle changes that are easily overlooked unless the examiner has a high index of suspicion for this disorder. Magnetic resonance imaging at this time will reveal marrow edema throughout the tarsal bones that are involved, and these findings generally overshadow the meager findings of plain radiographs. Stage I typically ends with the mechanical collapse of the foot.

Stage II is called the stage of coalescence, and is characterized by physiologic efforts to stabilize the foot through fibroblast proliferation and the formation of new bone. It is during this phase that exuberant fracture callus begins to form, often bridging multiple fragments of multiple bones. If immobilized, the foot tends to be less warm and swollen than during the acute stage. Stage III is called the stage of remodeling and healing. However, even several years after acute Charcot events, excessive motion and tarsal instability persists, which questions the existence of the third stage altogether.

A second system of classification of Charcot neuroarthropathy was described by Brodsky [15,16] and is based on the anatomical location of the injuries. Type I injuries involve the tarsometatarsal and the naviculocuneiform joints. This injury pattern tends to consolidate but is associated with a rocker bottom foot deformity and a significant incidence of midfoot ulceration. Type II injuries involve the major tarsal joints, including the subtalar, talonavicular and calcaneocuboid joints. These injuries are more difficult to treat because the resultant instability is multiplanar. Patients who develop this injury pattern require longer periods of time for consolidation and the prognosis for a functional foot is somewhat guarded. Type IIIa involves the ankle and is often associated with resorption of the talus and or navicular. Patients with this pattern of injury are unstable at the ankle and often develop severe frontal plane deformities with submalleolar ulcerations. Type IIIb injuries involve fractures through the body of the calcaneus, often associated with displacement of the tuberosity of the calcaneus by the pull of the triceps [15,16].

Schon [17] presented a scheme to describe midfoot injury patterns with an eye to developing treatment protocols for each specific type of injury. He also emphasized the importance of the stability of the lateral column of the foot in successful treatment of this condition. The Schon classification system included the Lisfranc, naviculocuneiform, perinavicular, and transverse tarsal patterns with subcategories to each pattern.

Sella and Barrette [18] introduced a classification system that described the findings in the medial column of Charcot neuroarthropathy. Clinical and radiographic findings were grouped into four stages (0–4), and treatment options were described for each stage.

The three stages described by Eichenholz represent the natural history of a Charcot event, without modification by treatment. Historically, Charcot events have been managed by off-loading, casting, and bracing, which did little to prevent deformity [19–21]. Over the past 10 years, a trend has developed toward operative intervention in the mature Charcot foot. The impetus for this change in direction lies in the desire to correct the foot deformity, thereby reducing the risk of plantar ulceration, which is the most common complication of foot collapse associated with Charcot neuroarthropathy [22–25].

Early diagnosis of an acute Charcot event

The primary goal in the treatment of any acute Charcot event is the recognition that such an event is occurring, even before the development of skeletal collapse. To recognize Charcot neuroarthropathy before the skeletal destruction occurs, one must maintain a high index of suspicion for the presence of the disorder. The presentation of unilateral edema, erythema, and warmth is often mistaken for cellulitis, and patients are mistakenly treated with a course of antibiotics. It is usually after the second cycle of antibiotics, because the first course was unsuccessful in resolving the patient's symptoms, when skeletal collapse becomes apparent. With a history of "cellulitis," the degenerative changes seen on radiographs are frequently interpreted as osteomyelitis. Unfortunately, treatment of these patients is then delayed while a great deal of time and resources are expended in the confirmation of the diagnosis of osteomyelitis. All too often, unnecessary ablative operations that produce a surgical specimen eventually refute the diagnosis of osteomyelitis.

It should be noted that a local infection in the foot is unlikely without a break in the skin's integrity, and hematogenous osteomyelitis in the diabetic population is far less common than osteomyelitis caused by direct penetration. Therefore, a patient with a swollen foot who has diabetic neuropathy and no portal of entry for an infection is much more likely to have acute Charcot neuroarthropathy than osteomyelitis. The differentiation of an acute Charcot event from osteomyelitis, in the presence of an ulcer, is somewhat more difficult. The use of bone scintigraphy, resonance imaging, and laboratory testing may prove helpful, but generally, with cellulitis and underlying acute osteomyelitis, a leucocytosis and a left shift would be expected. In osteomyelitis and acute Charcot events, erythrocyte sedimentation rates are elevated, but in the presence of osteomyelitis the values are generally higher, often at rates of 70 mm or greater per hour. Acute Charcot events also tend to involve several bones, whereas osteomyelitis in the midfoot or hindfoot is usually limited to the bone contiguous with the ulcer. Bone destruction in Charcot neuroarthropathy involving multiple bones is much greater than in an isolated osteomyelitis of a single tarsal bone. It is therefore reasonable to expect that patients who are experiencing an acute Charcot event are much more likely to demonstrate elevated serum alkaline phosphatase levels than patients with only chronic osteomyelitis [26,27].

Radiographic imaging, including technesium, labeled white cell scans, and sulfur colloid studies, although helpful, lack sufficient specificity to confidently distinguish an acute Charcot event from osteomyelitis in many cases. When doubt remains as to the presence of osteomyelitis, a bone biopsy may be helpful.

Management of Charcot neuroarthropathy

Traditionally, patients with Charcot neuroarthropathy in the acute phase are managed by immobilization. Regardless of the degree of deformity, the foot is usually casted until such time as the clinician feels that sufficient consolidation has been achieved to permit guarded weight-bearing. Skin thermography is often used as a criterion for the discontinuation of treatment. Deformities that develop as a result of collapse are accommodated with molded shoes, and more recently with custom-molded clamshell orthoses called Charcot restraint orthotic walkers (CROW). Unfortunately, many of these feet are difficult to accommodate, even with custom-molded shoes, and skin breakdown is common [28]. In the late 1980s and early 1990s, several reports of attempted reconstruction using techniques of internal fixation appeared. However, there were no statistically significant outcomes reported and, anecdotally, the reported morbidities and mortalities argued effectively against this approach [29–34].

Frykberg [35] reported a 25% incidence of acute Charcot events in the weight-bearing limbs of patients being treated for acute Charcot events in the other foot. Therefore, when an acute Charcot event is recognized it is important to mechanically protect the involved foot as well as the contralateral one. Because of this risk, it is prudent to protect the contralateral limb with a removable cast brace and to use a wheelchair during the period of treatment. A complicating feature of the treatment of acute Charcot neuroarthropathy is the absence of significant pain and the resultant and frequent lack of compliance of the patient. It is often difficult to convince patients with a well-developed work ethic and family responsibilities to adhere to the rules of strict non–weight-bearing in the absence of significant pain. The failure of conservative care is often due to the patient's inability to remain compliant during the period of treatment.

Current concepts in the treatment of Charcot neuroarthropathy

Charcot neuroarthropathy involving the hindfoot and midfoot often result in severe deformities of that extremity. This makes bracing and shoeing extremely difficult for a significant number of patients. In the presence of midfoot breakdowns, the cuboid and the navicular often become weight-bearing areas, leading to ulceration beneath these bones. Below-the-knee amputations for severe Charcot deformities and chronic ulcerations have historically been the definitive treatment for those patients who were unsuccessfully accommodated. More recently, attempts at reconstruction of the foot have been gaining popularity, due in large part to the use of multiplanar external fixators to maintain correction. Although the current literature is limited in reporting on these techniques, there are a number of centers where reconstruction of midfoot and hindfoot collapse are being treated aggressively.

The question that begs is why external fixation would succeed in maintaining correction when rigid internal fixation could not. The answer seems to be in the quality of the bone stock in patients with Charcot neuroarthropathy. Patients who have neuropathy demonstrate reduced bone stiffness and bone density [36–38]. Bone stiffness may be thought of as a measure of cortical integrity and bone density as a measure of how compact the cancellous bone is. In patients with reduced bone densities and stiffness, the application of interfragmental compression through lag screws and plates are likely doomed to failure. However, certain external fixation constructs, using tensioned thin wires inserted in multiple planes, seem to permit the application of interfragmental compression without the risk of implant loosening (Fig. 5). The use of threaded bone screws or transfixion pins in the tibia may be acceptable because of denser bone in the shank than in the foot, but their use in the tarsus should be used advisedly in this population.

Treatment of acute Charcot events

Ideally, a patient who is experiencing an acute Charcot event should be diagnosed during the early stages, before deformity develops. Patients who are diagnosed with a recent Charcot event present a challenging subset of individuals, particularly those whose foot has deformed. Do these individuals possess the potential to undergo acute reductions of their deformities? The traditional answer would be no. However, current thinking is redefining the limits of treatment. Acute Charcot events are coming to be regarded as acute pathological fracture/dislocation phenomena, which may well lend themselves to treatment by closed or open reduction.

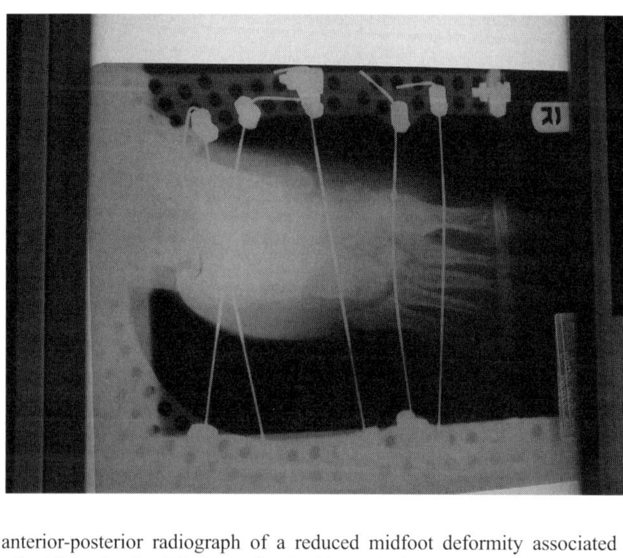

Fig. 5. An anterior-posterior radiograph of a reduced midfoot deformity associated with Charcot neuroarthropathy. The reduction is being maintained by multiple transosseous wires inserted in multiple planes. "Bent wire" technique was used to compress the metatarsals to the tarsus.

Because of the risk of skin breakdown under a cast, closed reduction, which requires manual pressure being applied to the foot during application, is usually contraindicated. The use of internal fixation in Charcot patients, including lag screws and plates, also carries a risk of failure because of osteopenic bone's inability to support screw threads. In addition, when internal fixation is used, the period of postoperative protection required before the patient may begin weight bearing is significantly extended. For these reasons, external fixation is being looked at critically as a viable alternative to cast immobilization or internal fixation. External fixation which uses transosseous thin wires in multiple planes is much less likely to loosen over time than are threaded half pins or centrally threaded transfixion pins, which rely more heavily on cortical stiffness and denser cancellous bone for their purchase (Figs. 1 and 6) [39–42].

In those patients whose foot has already collapsed, an assessment should be made as to whether they should be treated with immobilization and rest or whether an open reduction should be considered. The location of the collapse must be assessed and the inherent stability of the involved tarsal bones determined. Generally, midfoot disruption that results in a complete disassociation of the tarsometatarsal joints or plantar subluxation of the cuboid or navicular should be considered for operative intervention. Similarly, destruction of the ankle or subtalar joint that results in a significant varus or valgus deformity that would be difficult to brace and shoe should also be considered for operative treatment.

Open reduction

An open reduction of an acute Charcot event should be planned as one would plan any open reduction. However, the mechanical strength of the tarsal bones are compromised in these patients, and forceful maneuvers with bone skids and other instruments may result in further damage to the bones without necessarily reducing the deformity. If the deformity is not reducible, then consideration should be given to a correctional fusion of the involved joints. The use of lag screws and plates should generally be avoided, as implant loosening is common in patients with Charcot neuroarthropathy [43,44]. The limited use of screws, in conjunction with external fixation, may be a viable option. An external fixator will mechanically bridge the arthrodesis site and neutralize stress within the tarsus. A multiplanar external fixation construct alone can provide adequate interfragmental stabilization. This may be accomplished by the using a "bent wire technique." This involves the transosseous passage of a thin wire through a segment of the foot distal to the site of arthrodesis. The wires are then attached to the external fixator at either end, at points proximal to where the wire emerges from the foot. As the wire is tensioned to the frame the wire is forced to straighten and as it does the segment of the foot to which it is attached is pulled back and impacted against the proximal segment (Fig. 5).

Acute Charcot events involving the ankle are more difficult to treat. If the talus becomes avascular, as is often the case with Brodsky IIIa lesions, then anatomical reduction is no longer an option. Astragalectomy and tibiocalcaneal arthrodesis should be considered in these patients [45]. However, rates of nonunion in these

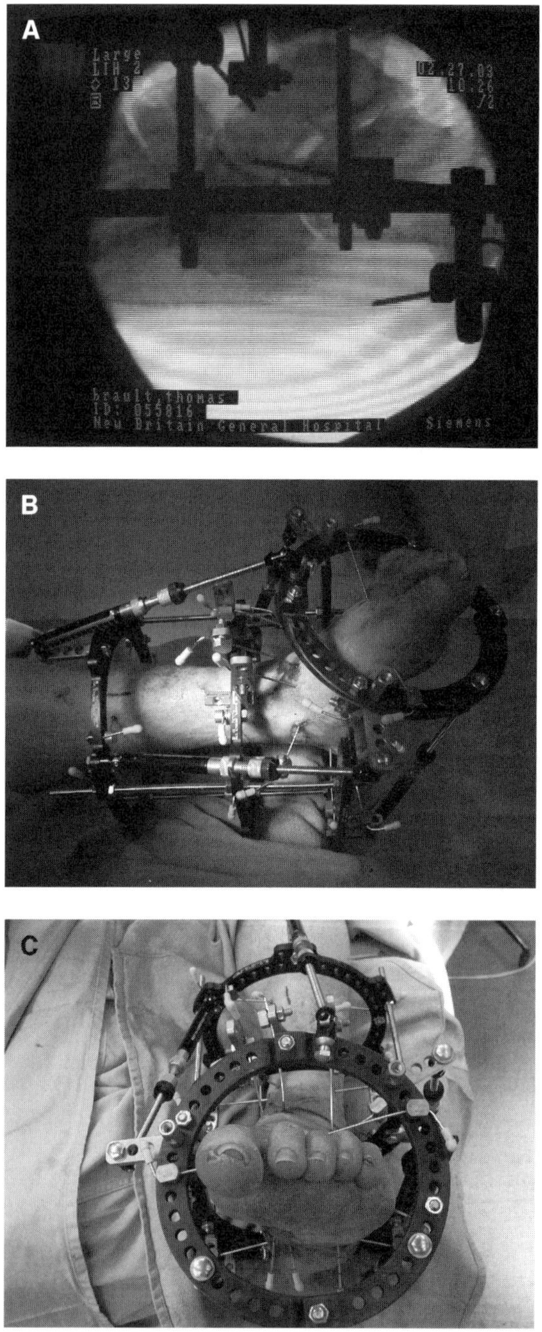

Fig. 6. (*A–C*) An acute Charcot of the midfoot treated with the application of an Ilizarov frame for closed reduction by distraction.

patients are high. Fusing the calcaneocuboid joint will help to stabilize the lateral column and reduce the likelihood of the tibia wedging itself through the midfoot. The use of intramedullary nails for fixation of tibiocalcaneal fusions has become popular, and the development of second-generation devices that apply axial compression is a clear improvement over earlier designs; however, it has recently been shown that intramedullary locking nails are not as stable as multiplanar external fixation. An external fixator may be used as an adjunct to an intramedullary nail [46].

Closed reduction

In selected patients, where the time between injury and collapse is less than 20 weeks, closed reduction of the foot may be attempted. This is facilitated by the use of a circular external fixator. Forceful manipulation of the foot risks injury to the soft tissue envelope and the long-term use of casts certainly increases that risk. In patients with midfoot disruptions whose interval between event and collapse is less than 2 weeks, the use of gradual distraction by an Ilizarov frame may be contemplated. The design of such a frame would require the leg, and tarsal bones proximal to the lesion, to be included in a "boot." The forefoot is then engaged by an encircling ring and several thin wires. The forefoot ring is then attached to the boot by several adjustable connecting rods, and distraction of that ring is commenced at a gradual rate of approximately 1 mm per day. By varying the rate of lengthening of the connecting rods, the forefoot and the distal ring may be deflected into plantarflexion, adduction, or adduction as needed. If at any time closed reduction is not producing the desired result, then a decision to convert to an open reduction can be made.

Treatment of chronic Charcot deformities

The goal of treating a patient with a Charcot deformity is to avoid skin breakdown and restore a stable foot. In patients with midfoot deformities, the use of extradepth shoes and accommodative inlays may be sufficient in patients with minimal deformity and a stable midfoot. Where the deformity is more severe or where the midfoot is unstable, then the use of molded shoes should be considered. In some patients, the use of patellar tendon bearing orthoses may be required to prevent plantar ulceration.

If plantar ulceration occurs, despite attempts at accommodation, consideration should be given to either an ostectomy or midfoot fusion. This may be performed in conjunction with a soft tissue reconstruction [47]. Midfoot ulcers beneath the lateral column have a higher incidence of recurrence than do those beneath the medial column, when treated by simple ostectomy [48]. Therefore, lateral midfoot ulcers associated with a Charcot deformity should be treated with arthrodesis and soft tissue reconstruction.

The rocker bottom appearance associated with Charcot collapse is usually seen with a transverse plane component. Multiplanar wedge resection may be performed and held in reduction with an external fixator (Fig. 7). This avoids the use of implanted metal in areas of bone with a history of chronic ulceration and inflammation. In addition, contraction of the triceps surae is a common finding associated with a midfoot collapse and will likely require a lengthening of the triceps at the time of reconstruction to prevent recurrent plantar breakdown (Fig. 8) [49–51].

Patients with significant varus or valgus ankle deformities may be considered as candidates for triple arthrodesis, ankle fusion, or a tibiocalcaneal arthrodesis. Because the talus is often avascular in cases involving disruption of the subtalar joint, it may be prudent to resect the talus and fuse the tibia directly to the calcaneus. The use of locking intramedullary nails with or without supplementation by an external fixator would be the fixation of choice. Arthrodesing operations in the Charcot population carries a significant risk for nonunion. However, clinical

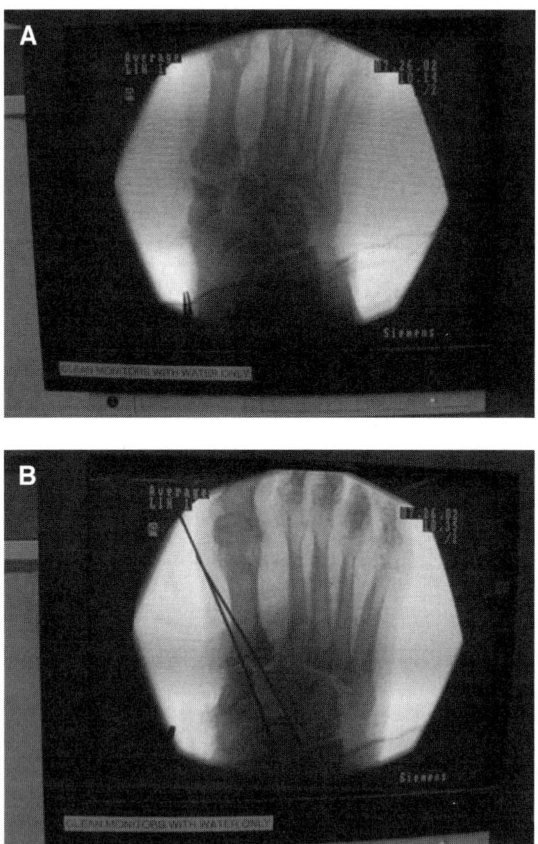

Fig. 7. (*A,B*) Anteroposterior radiograph of a foot before and after a medially based wedge was removed from the lesser tarsus for the correction of a chronic Charcot deformity.

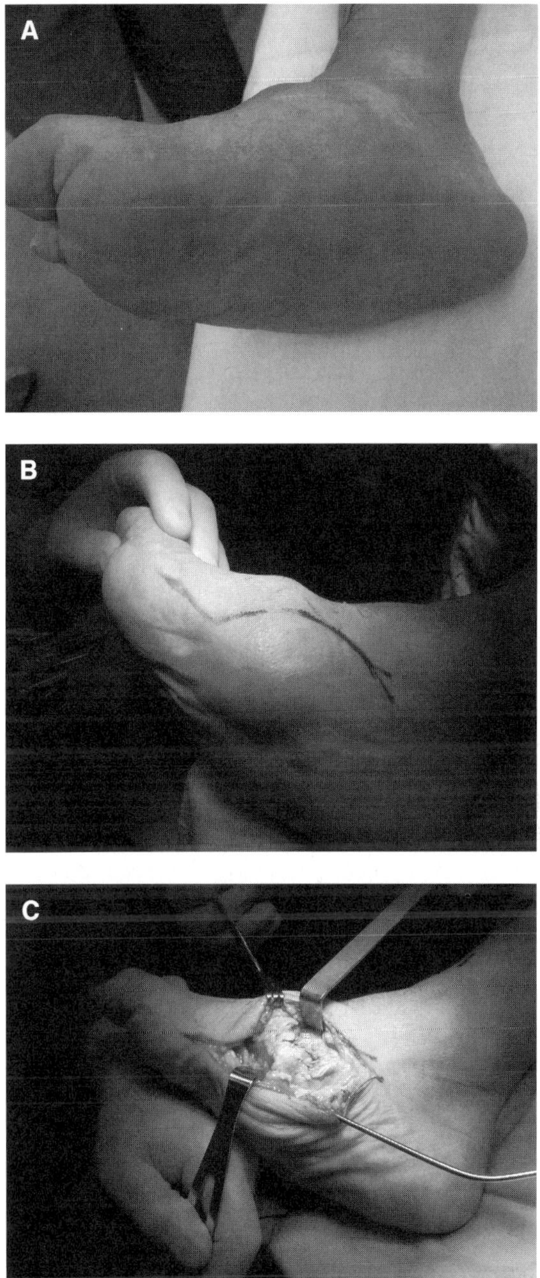

Fig. 8. Correction of a chronic Charcot deformity. (*A*) Preoperative appearance of the foot. (*B*) Incision placement. (*C*) Exposure of the medial tarsus. (*D*) The Ilizarov fixator in place.

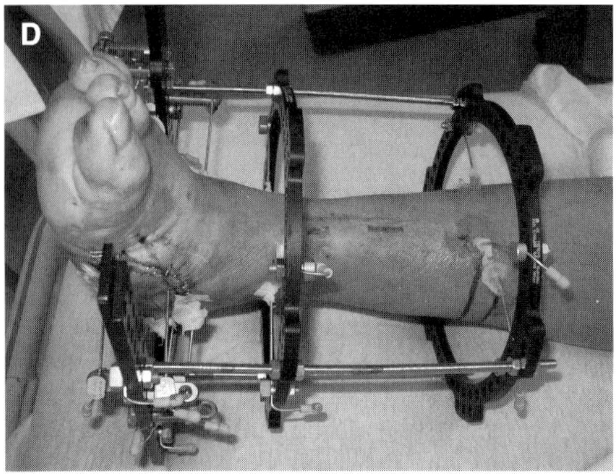

Fig. 8 (*continued*).

success in obtaining a painless and stable foot is not dependant on radiographic evidence of fusion [52].

Summary

Charcot neuroarthropathy is a complex sequela of neuropathies associated with diabetes mellitus, syringomyelia, alcoholism, and other disorders. The treatment of deformities associated with Charcot neuroarthropathy is evolving from a passive approach to one in which an earlier recognition of the emergence of the event permits an avoidance of deformity. As the understanding of the etiology and natural history of Charcot neuroarthropathy deepens, it has become apparent that many of the deformities that do develop may be reconstructed expeditiously by the surgeon with a thorough understanding of the diabetic foot and experience in the use of external fixation.

References

[1] Kelly M. William Musgrave's De arthritide symptomatica (1703): his description of neuropathic arthritis. Bull Hist Med 1963;37:372–6.
[2] Charcot JM. Sur quelques arthropaties qui paraissent deponder d'une lesion du cerveau ou de la moele epiniere. Arch Physiol Norm Pathol 1868;1:161–71.
[3] Jordan WR. Neuritic manifestations in diabetes mellitus. Arch Intern Med 1936;57:307–12.
[4] Armstrong DG, Todd WF, Lavery LA, et al. The natural history of acute Charcot's arthropathy in a diabetic foot specialty clinic. Diabet Med 1997;14:357–63.
[5] Schon LC, Easley ME, Weinfeld SB. Charcot neuroarthropathy of the foot and ankle. Clin Orthop 1998;349:116–31.
[6] Brower AC, Allman RM. Pathogenesis of the neurotrophic joint: neurotraunatic vs. neurovascular. Radiology 1981;139:349–54.
[7] Johnson JTH. Neurotrophic fractures and joint injuries. Pathogenesis and rationale of prevention and treatment. J Bone Joint Surg 1967;49:1–30.

[8] Slowman-Kovacs SD, Braunstein EM, Brandt KD. Rapidly progressive Charcot arthropathy following minor joint trauma in patients with diabetic neuropathy. Arthritis Rheum 1990;33: 412–7.
[9] Edmonds ME, Clarke MB, Newton S, et al. Increased uptake of bone radiopharmaceutical in diabetic neuropathy. Q J Med 1985;57:843–55.
[10] Gough A, Abraha H, Purewal TS, et al. Measurement of markers of osteoclast and osteoblast activity in patients with acute and chronic diabetic Charcot neuroarthropathy. Diabet Med 1997; 14:527–31.
[11] Brooks AP. The neuropathic foot in diabetes. Part II: Charcot's neuroarthropathy. Diabet Med 1986;3:116–8.
[12] Stevens MJ, Edmonds ME, Foster AVM, et al. Paradoxical blood flow responses in the diabetic neuropathic foot: an assessment of the contribution of vascular denervation and microangiopathy. Diabet Med 1992;9:49–54.
[13] Jirkovska A, Kasalicky P, Boucek P, et al. Calcaneal ultrasonometry in patients with Charcot osteoarthropathy and its relationship with densitometry in the lumbar spine and femoral neck and with markers of bone turnover. Diabet Med 2001;18:495–500.
[14] Eichenholtz SN. Charcot joints. Springfield (IL): C.C. Thomas; 1966.
[15] Brodsky JW, Rouse AM. Exostectomy for symptomatic bony prominences in diabetic Charcot feet. Clin Orthop 1993;296:21–6.
[16] Brodsky JW. The diabetic foot. In: Mann RA, Coughlin M, editors. Surgery of the foot and ankle. St. Louis (MO): Mosby; 1993. p. 925–53.
[17] Schon LC, Easley ME, Weinfeld SB. Charcot neuroarthropathy of the foot and ankle. Clin Orthop 1998;349:116–31.
[18] Sella EJ, Barrette C. Staging of Charcot neuroarthropathy along the medial column of the foot in the diabetic patient. J Foot Ankle Surg 1999;38:34–40.
[19] Myerson M, Papa J, Eaton K, et al. The total-contact cast for management of neuropathic plantar ulceration of the foot. J Bone Joint Surg 1992;74:261–9.
[20] Morgan JM, Biehl WC, Wagner FW. Management of neuropathic arthropathy with the Charcot restraint orthotic walker. Clin Orthop 1993;296:58–63.
[21] Armstrong DG, Lavery LA. Elevated peak plantar pressures in patients who have Charcot arthropathy. J Bone Joint Surg 1998;80:365–9.
[22] Early JS, Hansen ST. Surgical reconstruction of the diabetic foot: a salvage approach for midfoot collapse. Foot Ankle Int 1996;17:325–30.
[23] Papa JS, Myerson MS, Girard P. Salvage with arthrodesis in intractable diabetic neuropathic arthropathy of the foot and ankle. J Bone Joint Surg 1993;75:1056–66.
[24] Stuart MJ, Morrey BF. Arthrodesis of the diabetic neuropathic ankle joint. Clin Orthop 1990;253: 209–11.
[25] Sammarco GJ, Conti SF. Surgical treatment of neuroarthropathic foot deformity. Foot Ankle Int 1998;19:102–9.
[26] Kaleta JL, Fleischli JW, Reilly CH. The diagnosis of osteomyelitis in diabetes using erythrocyte sedimentation rate: a pilot study. J Am Podiatr Med Assoc 2001;91:445–50.
[27] Peters KM, Rosendahl T, Heller KD, et al. Osteocalcin levels in chronic osteomyelitis. Arch Orthop Trauma Surg 1994;114:53–5.
[28] Cundy TF, Edmonds ME, Watkins PJ. Osteopenia and metatarsal fractures in diabetic neuropathy. Diabet Med 1985;2:461–4.
[29] Bono JV, Roger DJ, Jacobs RL. Surgical arthrodesis of the neuropathic foot: a salvage procedure. Clin Orthop 1993;296:14–20.
[30] Fabrin J, Larsen K, Holstein PE. Long-term follow-up in diabetic Charcot feet with spontaneous onset. Diabetes Care 2000;23:796–800.
[31] Faglia E, Favales F, Morabito A. New ulceration, new major amputation, and survival rates in diabetic subjects hospitalized for foot ulceration from 1990 to 1993. Diabetes Care 2001;24:78–83.
[32] Pinzur MS, Kelikian A. Charcot ankle fusion with a retrograde locked intramedullary nail. Foot Ankle Int 1997;18:699–704.

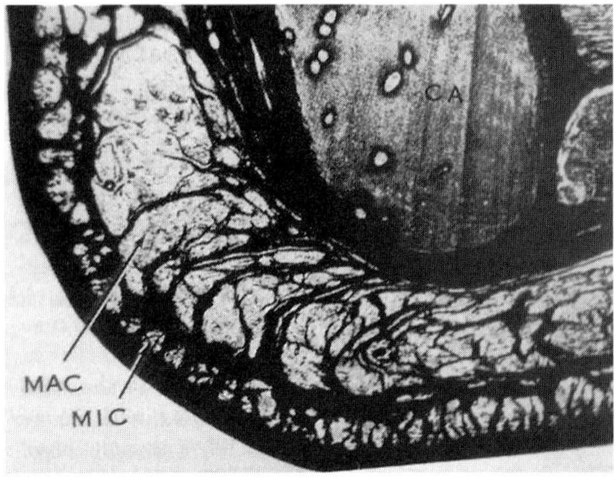

Fig. 1. A cross-section through a fetal foot. The mooring ligaments and columnar fat bodies can be seen.

ligaments are a series of bands that secure the deep layer of the dermis to the deep fascia, and it is the presence of these ligaments that resist shear. The superficial layer of the plantar fascia attaches to the dermis at the junction of the plantar arch and the ball of the foot. When the foot is loaded and the plantar fascia is under tension, the plantar skin is stabilized in part by the plantar fascia. The recruitment of mooring ligaments during weight bearing is dependant on the magnitude of the shearing force that is applied and the surface area of the foot that is under load. As both of these variables increase, the number of mooring ligaments under tension will increase proportionally.

When wounds on the plantar surface of the foot are allowed to heal by secondary intention, the resultant scars possesses none of the resilient characteristics of the lost tissue, and so significant strain builds at the margin of scar and skin during weight-bearing activities. Scar tissue on the bottom of the foot is unable to move in concert with the surrounding soft tissue and so friction develops over the scar, resulting in blister formation and eventual callus. In the insensate foot, the callus eventually produces pressure necrosis of the skin beneath, leading to the formation of a new ulcer.

As an alternative to healing by secondary intention, numerous techniques have been described which may be used to resurface defects on the weight-bearing and non–weight-bearing surfaces of the foot. The advantage of these reconstructive techniques over healing by secondary intention is that their tissue properties more closely resemble the tissue properties of the lost tissues, so that movement of the flap will more closely resemble the movement of the surrounding soft tissue during weight-bearing activities. This prevents strain from developing at the margins.

Closure of plantar wounds by primary intention significantly reduces the duration of treatment and, subsequently, the expense of treating a foot wound. The costs associated with the treatment of chronic wounds are significant in terms of professional care, hospital charges, and outpatient costs of dressing materials and nursing visits. There are also psychological and social burdens that must be borne by the patient and his or her family during the course of treatment for a chronic wound. Those burdens obviously increase with the duration of the treatment [2–4].

The application of the principles and techniques of plastic surgery to the treatment of the foot began in the 1980s, and the integration of these techniques into the armamentarium of the foot and ankle surgeon has progressed quickly [5–8]. This article will provide an introduction to the principles and methods of soft tissue reconstruction of the diabetic foot.

Skin grafting

Skin grafting is an extremely effective technique for providing fast and easy coverage of wounds. Skin grafts are either full thickness or partial thickness, and each has specific characteristics. Full-thickness skin grafts are harvested by excision and include the epidermis, dermis, and the skin adnexa, such as sweat glands, hair follicles, and oil glands. Full-thickness grafts, when applied to a wound, will prevent the wound from undergoing further contraction. Full-thickness skin grafts are usually harvested from areas where there is a skin redundancy, such as from the flexor surfaces of joints, such as the wrist, over the sinus tarsi, or the inguinal fold. Full-thickness skin grafts may also be harvested from the lateral thigh. When a skin graft is taken, the donor site is closed primarily. Skin grafts should only be applied to areas that are surgically clean and free of necrotic tissue. Skin grafts will fail if the wound to which they are being applied is colonized or frankly infected, or if there is active bleeding or transudation, which can lead to a hematoma or seroma and prevent adherence of the graft to the bed.

Skin grafts may be applied to subcutaneous fat, tendon sheath, and in some cases freshly decorticated cancellous bone, although these grafts tend to be unstable. The application of skin grafts to bare tendon or fascia, which is avascular, will usually not be able to sustain viability of the graft. It is sometimes possible to generate granulation over tendon or fascia by using meticulous wound care, exogenous growth factors, and laboratory-engineered tissue. Once a healthy layer of granulation has formed over the exposed surface of the tendon or fascia, skin grafting becomes a viable option.

Split-thickness skin grafts are harvested tangentially and include the epidermis and, depending on the thickness, elements of the dermis. A dermatome is used to perform the harvest, and most modern dermatomes allow for graft thicknesses of between 5/1000 and 30/1000 of an inch. Unlike full-thickness skin grafts, split-thickness skin grafts when applied to a wound do not completely prevent further wound contraction. The site of harvest is covered postoperatively with petroleum jelly-impregnated gauze, which is allowed to slough as epitheliazation progresses beneath it.

When skin grafts are harvested, the blood supply to the graft is disrupted, so the graft should be applied to the recipient site as expeditiously as possible. Survival of the flap is dependant on its rapid revascularization. Inosculation of skin grafts by

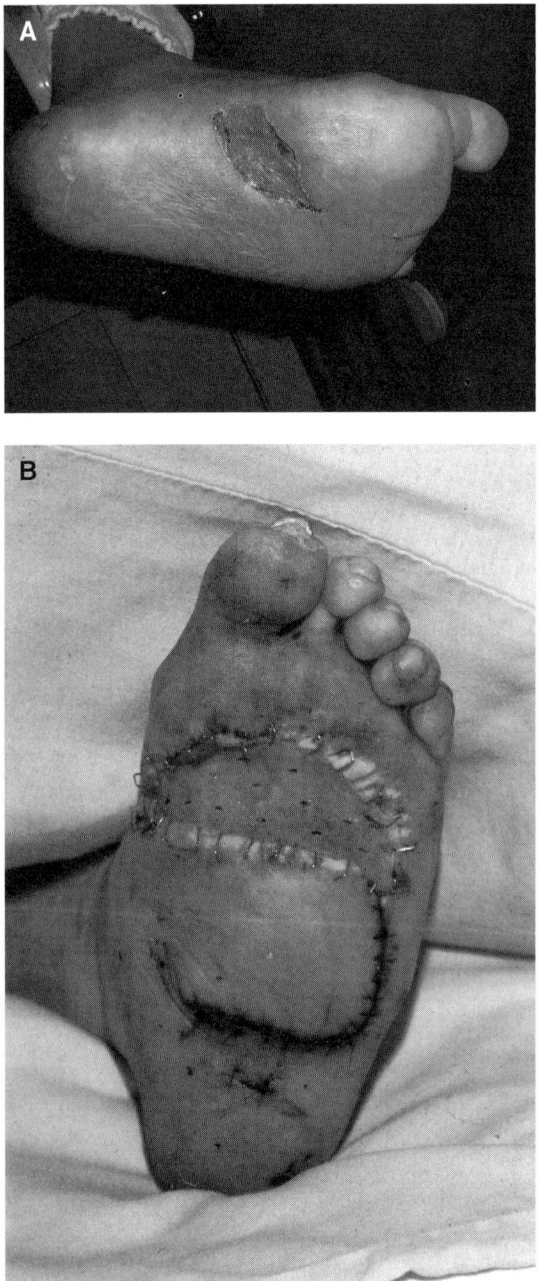

Fig. 2. (*A*) A split-thickness skin graft covering a defect in the instep. (*B*) A split thickness skin graft used to cover a donor site from a transposition flap.

vascular buds usually begins by the fifth postoperative day, and proceeds until venous drainage of the graft has been established, usually by the second week [9–11].

During the first postoperative week, the graft's viability is maintained by a process of diffusion known as plasmatic imbibition, until inosculation of the graft has been established. During the first 48 hours, fibrin is laid down between the graft and the bed, which helps to anchor the graft to the donor site. To prevent disruption of this tenuous anchorage, a nonadherent dressing, which protects the graft from shear during the immediate postoperative period, is applied. It is axiomatic that thin, split-thickness grafts "take" better than do full-thickness grafts, because the thinness of the graft allows for easier imbibition and a more rapid inosculation. In the diabetic foot this is a major consideration.

In treating defects in the diabetic foot, split-thickness skin grafts are used frequently in non–weight-bearing areas or to cover donor sites of locally raised flaps (Fig. 2). The use of skin grafts in areas that are subjected to significant stress is to be avoided [12].

Local random flaps

Local flaps are extremely useful for reconstruction of diabetic foot wounds. They allow for the transfer of adjacent tissue with similar properties to provide coverage. These flaps provide durability in this extremely complex patient population [13–15]. A limiting factor to the success of any reconstructive procedure in the diabetic patient is adequate perfusion of the foot. Therefore, a thorough assessment of the perfusion of the tissues is required before considering soft tissue reconstruction.

In developing local plantar flaps, the dissection provides ample exposure to underlying osseous deformities and pockets of necrotic or frankly infected bone, allowing for a more thorough debridement than would a dorsal incision. The coverage that these flaps provide allows for primary closure of the wound and usually prevents scar contracture and junctional fibrosis, which is commonly seen when wounds are allowed to granulate and heal by secondary intention [16]. Closure of chronic diabetic wounds by local flaps may be performed at the time of debridement, or the flap may be delayed, depending on wound conditions at the time [17].

A local flap may be defined as an area of tissue, adjacent to a defect, which is mobilized and inserted into that defect to provide closure. These flaps are vascularized by random blood vessels that penetrate the flap to provide arterial and venous supply [18]. Local flaps are typically based on geometric designs and include epidermis, dermis, and subcutaneous tissue, but in certain situations can be designed to include fascia and muscle. Local flaps may be used to cover bone, tendon, and underlying subcutaneous tissue.

There is a subset of local skin flaps that are useful for closure of diabetic foot wounds [17]. These designs may be categorized by the nature of their movement from their donor site to their recipient site. The three categories of flap movement are advancement, transposition, and rotation. Each movement permits a number of flap designs that provide coverage of a plantar defect. The type of flap selected is often dependant on the nature of the neurovascular supply to the area of the foot that contains the defect. The design of most flaps used on the sole of the foot have been borrowed from other anatomic areas of the body, such as the hand and face, which have inherently greater mobility than does the sole of the foot. The application of these flaps to the foot is somewhat limited by the unique properties of the weight-bearing soft tissue and their lack of mobility. As a result of these properties, there are several designs that have been found to be more useful than other local flaps for diabetic foot reconstruction.

The plantar surface of the foot may be divided into the forefoot, midfoot, and hindfoot, with the skin in each area receiving its neurovascular supply in slightly different patterns. The choice of a particular flap is often based in part on these "random" patterns of neurovascular supply [19]. The rules that govern the development of random flaps in other anatomic areas, such as the face and hand, do not always apply when reconstructing the sole of the foot. In the foot, there is often underlying bone pathology, which is addressed through ostectomy. Resection of a portion of a bone segment often creates laxity within the overlying soft tissues, permitting flap movement that would be unavailable without bone resection.

Relaxed skin tension lines and lines of maximal extensibility should be taken into consideration when planning flaps. A line of maximal extensibility typically runs perpendicular to the relax skin tension lines, and relaxed skin tension lines run perpendicular to the axis of movement of the joint or tendon. Incisions that are typically placed parallel to the relaxed skin tension lines tend to heal with less scarring because wound contraction does not interfere with joint movement. However, the rules of relaxed skin tension lines and lines of maximal extensibility can often be ignored when bony realignment procedures are performed simultaneously.

Flap viability is based on the mobility and elasticity of the flap and its ability to relocate without tension. The tissue being harvested for reconstruction should be equal to or greater in durability and mobility than the original skin of the recipient site [20]. Weight-bearing plantar tissue should ideally be replaced with other weight-bearing plantar tissue. If donor sites require split thickness skin grafting they should be limited to the arch and other areas of low functional demand.

The blood supply to these flaps is derived from three anatomic patterns: a cutaneous artery, a musculocutaneous perforating artery, or a septocutaneous perforator. Blood vessels radiate, from fixed areas where tissues are anchored, to more mobile areas of tissue. Where there is mobility between tissue planes over a wide area, large flaps are frequently available for transfer [21]. It follows then that the safest design of a local flap is where the axis of the flap is displaced along the direction of the greatest mobility or lines of maximum extensibility, as determined by the pinch test, and toward the next dominant perforating artery.

It has been demonstrated that from the heel to the base of the metatarsals there exists an extensive subcutaneous neurovascular plexus, the result of colaterallization between the maleollar and tarsal arteries with perforators from the medial and lateral plantar arteries. Therefore, in the heel and midfoot, flaps can be safely raised with a transverse lie [19]. Thc plantar surface of the forefoot receives its neurovascular supply from perforators that arise from the plantar metatarsal arteries and nerves and pierce between the slips of the plantar fascia. At the subcutaneous level and at the dermis, they arborize to form a rich vascular plexus. Because local flaps in this area are supplied from pedicles oriented from deep to superficial, their orientation is determined by dimensional considerations rather than vascular ones.

To ensure viability, surgical techniques for the development of flaps must be meticulous. Atraumatic handling of the tissue, using skin hooks and sharp dissection, is essential in avoiding marginal flap necrosis. Flaps are sutured with simple nylon, typically 4-0, and deep sutures should be avoided at all costs. Following excision of the defect and removal of all necrotic tissue, the wound should be irrigated with 4 L normal saline, the foot should be redraped, and the surgical team should change gloves.

Local flaps are created by undermining in the suprafascial plane, releasing the tethering effects of the mooring ligaments. The extent of undermining should be only as extensive as necessary to permit movement, as excessive dissection may jeopardize a flap's viability. Vessels that perforate the flap should be preserved, and hemostasis should be achieved with a fine point cautery. Hematomas can be devastating and cause necrosis of the entire flap. All dead spaces should be drained.

The postoperative care of each local flap is extremely important and requires close observation. Light dressings, which are nonconstrictive, should be used, and strict adherence to a period of non–weight-bearing and elevation is essential. Evaluation of a flap postoperatively should include evaluation of the capillary refill. Patients who have end-stage renal disease and are on dialysis typically require 4 weeks of strict non–weight-bearing before their sutures are removed. Each patient who undergoes reconstruction will heal at his or her own pace, and sutures should not be removed prematurely.

Advancement flaps

Advancement flaps involve linear movement of skin and subcutaneous tissue from a donor site to a recipient site. Advancement flaps have proven to be of great value in closing wounds on the plantar surface of the forefoot. Because the blood supply to the skin in this region is derived from a series of perforators, which arise from the plantar metatarsal vessels and arborize into a subcutaneous and subdermal plexus, islands of skin and subcutaneous tissue can be created and moved in any direction within the limits of the extensibility of the perforating vessels. A careful release of the mooring ligaments and preservation of the vascular pedicles will permit surface movement of up to 1.5 cm in any direction. For defects greater in size, two flaps of similar dimensions may be designed to move toward each other to resurface such a defect. These flaps are typically designed so that their trailing edge is tear drop in shape, so the donor site may be closed primarily in a V to Y fashion (Fig. 3).

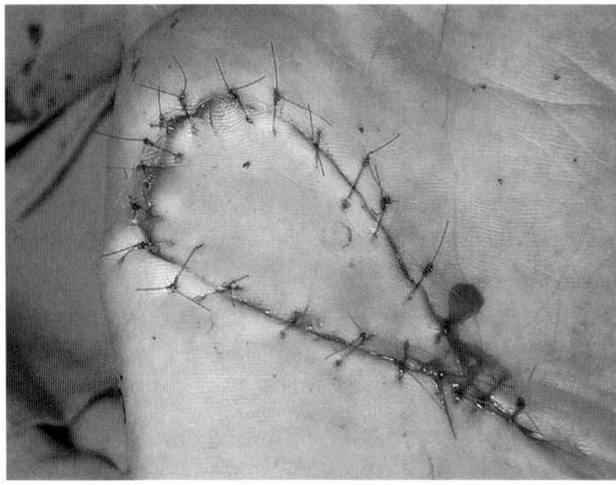

Fig. 3. A V-Y advancement flap on the sole of the foot.

Rotation flaps

Rotation flaps are preferred for closure of midfoot wounds, especially those associated with a Charcot deformity. Rotation flaps pivot around a point and move through an arc. Rotation flaps can be subfascial or suprafascial (Fig. 4) [22]. Rotation flaps can be elevated from the non–weight-bearing arch and rotated to weight-bearing areas such as the heel. These flaps allow for broad exposure to the underlying collapse of the midtarsus and Lisfranc's joint and provide easy access for ostectomy of fusion. A rotation flap is considered an excellent option for closure of a circular or triangular defect of the plantar surface of the foot. An arcuate-shaped flap is designed so that the leading tip of the flap will rotate around the circumference of the circle on which the defect lies. To ensure closure of the donor site, the flap should have a radius five to eight times the width of the defect. The major movement is in the rotation of the flap. Secondary movements of the adjacent or surrounding skin toward the flap are made possible by undermining the recipient site. Key sutures are placed along the closing edge of the flap. Primary closure of a rotation flap usually results in a "dog ear" along the radius and is resolved by triangular excision.

Transposition flaps

Transposition flaps allow for coverage of defects in adjacent territories and are based on a rectangular design. These flaps are tongue-like in shape and generally have narrower bases than do rotation flaps. The surface area of a transposition flap is less than the surface area of a rotation flap covering a defect of the same size. Transposition flaps are also more likely to require split-thickness skin grafts, especially in the plantar arch region, to close their donor sites than are rotation flaps. Transposition flaps are capable of covering larger wounds in the plantar hindfoot than will rotation flaps, because the coverage of the donor site by a split-thickness skin graft augments the total surface area (Fig. 5). A number of

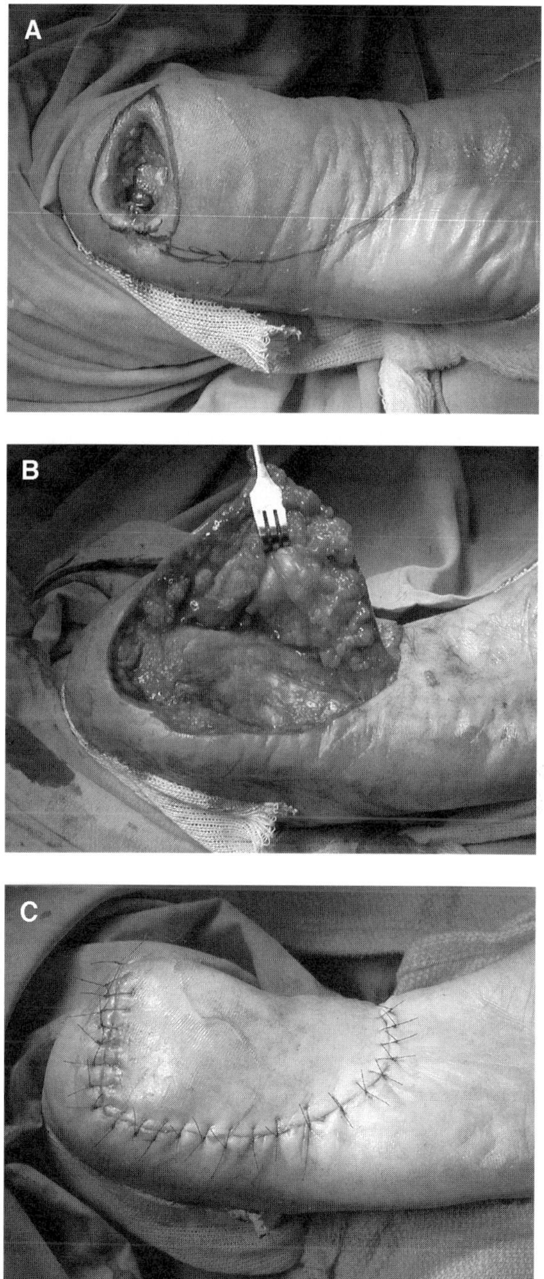

Fig. 4. A rotation flap to cover a plantar heel ulcer. (*A*) The ulcer is excised and an arc of rotation is planned. (*B*) A suprafascial flap is raised. (*C*) The flap is inset and the incision closed primarily.

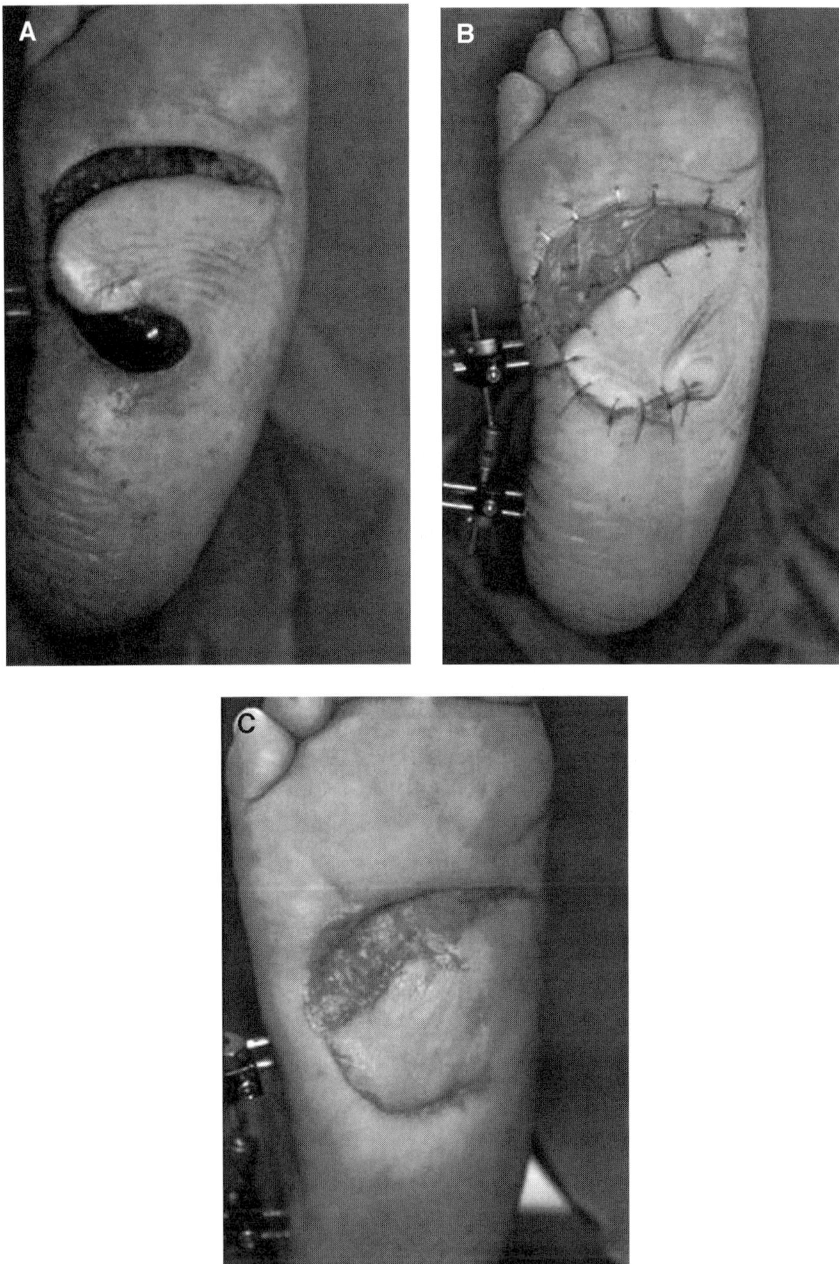

Fig. 5. A transposition flap. (*A*) A tongue-shaped flap is raised from the instep. (*B*) The flap is inset and the donor site covered with a split-thickness skin graft. (*C*) A viable flap and complete "take" of the skin graft.

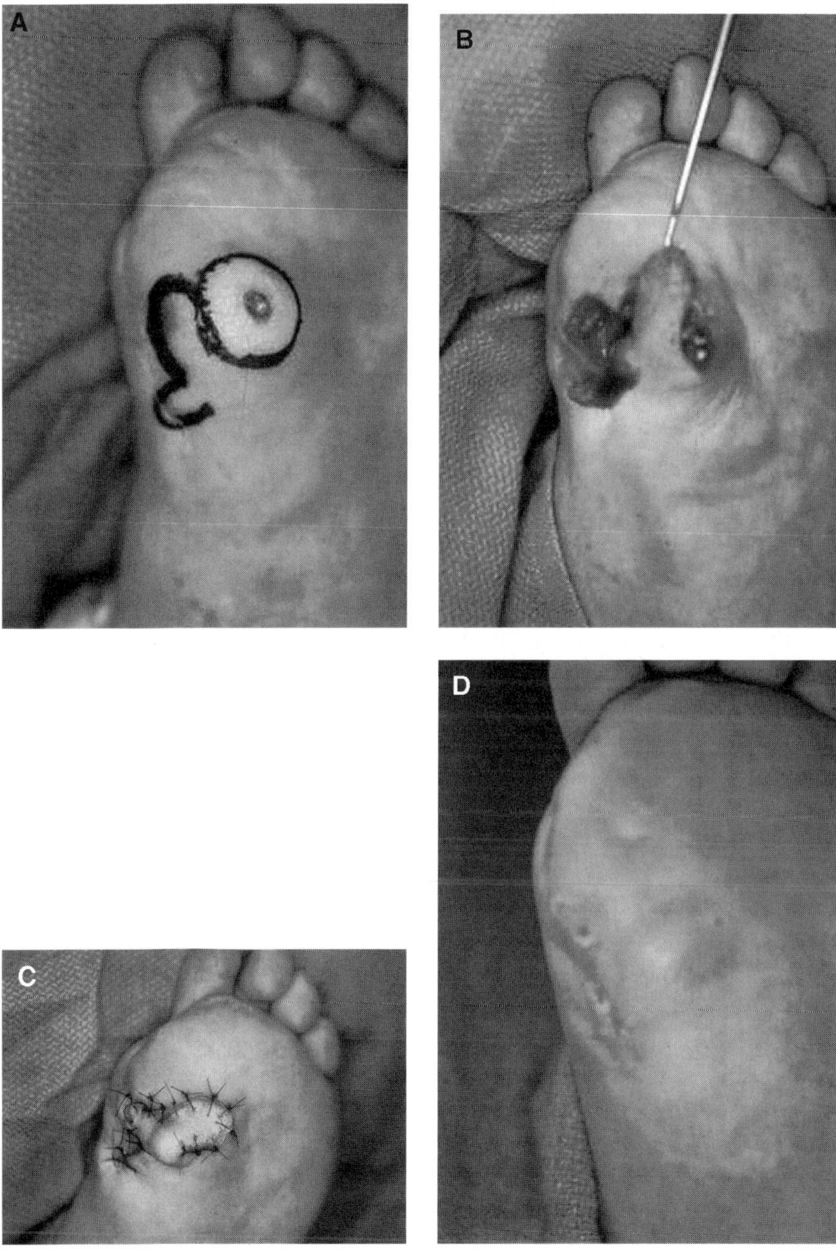

Fig. 6. A bilobed flap. (*A*) Planning of the flap. Note that the near lobe is 0.75 of the width of the defect and the far flap is 0.5. (*B*) After excision of the ulcer the flap has been undermined and transposed. (*C*) After inset of the flap. (*D*) The appearance of the flap at 3 months.

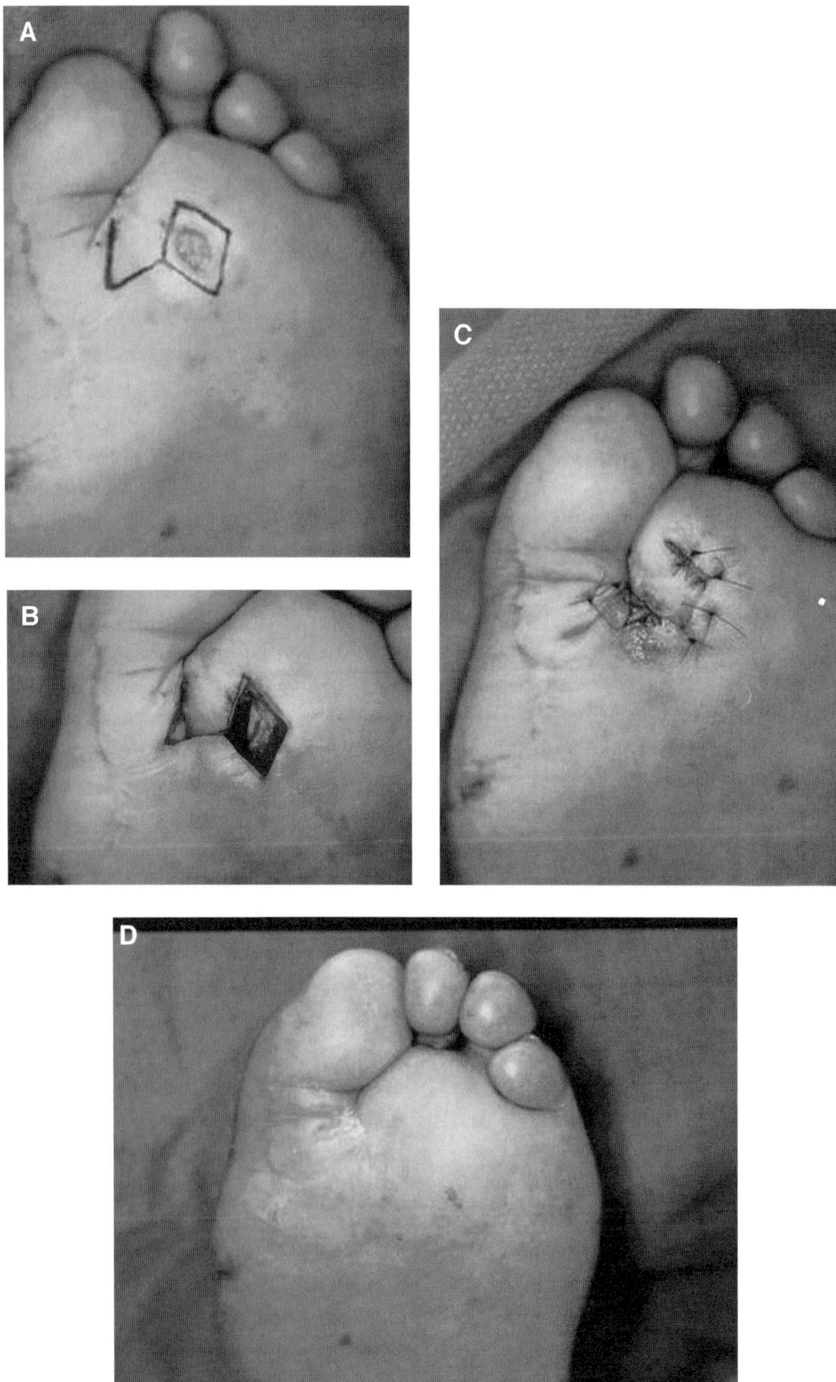
A
B
C
D

modifications to the standard transposition flap have been described and many have found use in the foot.

Bilobed flaps

The bilobed flap was originally described by Esser and later modified by Zimany [23]. This design consists of two lobes that are separated by an angle and share a common pedicle (Fig. 6). It is designed to incrementally move more skin over a larger distance than would be possible with a simple transposition flap, and typically works well in regions were skin mobility and elasticity is sometimes limited. The lobe of the flap adjacent to the defect is used to close the original defect, while the second lobe closes the first flap's donor site. The second flap donor site is then closed primarily as an elipse. Typically the lobes are designed to be 90 degrees from the defect and from each other [8]. Generally, the first lobe should be approximately 75% of the width of the original defect; the width of the second lobe should be 50% of the original defect. The rotating base should be the only area undermined. These flaps allow for exposure of the underlying bone and are often used in the plantar surface of the forefoot. It can be used for coverage of defects between 1 cm and 3 sq cm.

Rhomboid flaps

The rhomboid or Limberg flap is another workhorse for closure of diabetic forefoot wounds [24,25]. The wound is converted to a rhomboid shape with acute angles of 60 degrees and obtuse angles of 120 degrees. There are four quadrants from which a flap may be raised [26]. Because of the geometry of the flap, the choice of four potential flaps makes this technique useful and also allows for broad exposure of underlying bone deformities. The orientation of the flap should be ideally raised within the relaxed skin tension lines (Fig. 7).

Double-Z rhomboid flaps

The double-Z rhomboid flap integrates two Z-plasties into its design. This type of flap is typically used to correct a diamond-shaped defect [27]. This flap is extremely useful for forefoot ulcerations, particularly those that are close to the edge of the foot. This flap was originally described as a rhomboid to W flap. The technique for development of this flap includes two sets of parallel lines drawn to complete a 60 and 120 degree rhombus (Fig. 8A). Two Z-plasties are then extended from the opposite acute angles of the rhombus, such that their central lines are continuations of the original two parallel lines of the rhombus. The flaps are then transposed as in a Z-plasty, resulting in an incision shaped like two Z's aligned end to end (Fig. 8B).

Fig. 7. Rhomboid flap. (*A*) Flap planning. Note that the dimensions of the flap are the same as the planned defect. (*B*) Excision of the ulcer and mobilization of the flap. (*C*) Closure of the wound and donor site. (*D*) Appearance after 3 months.

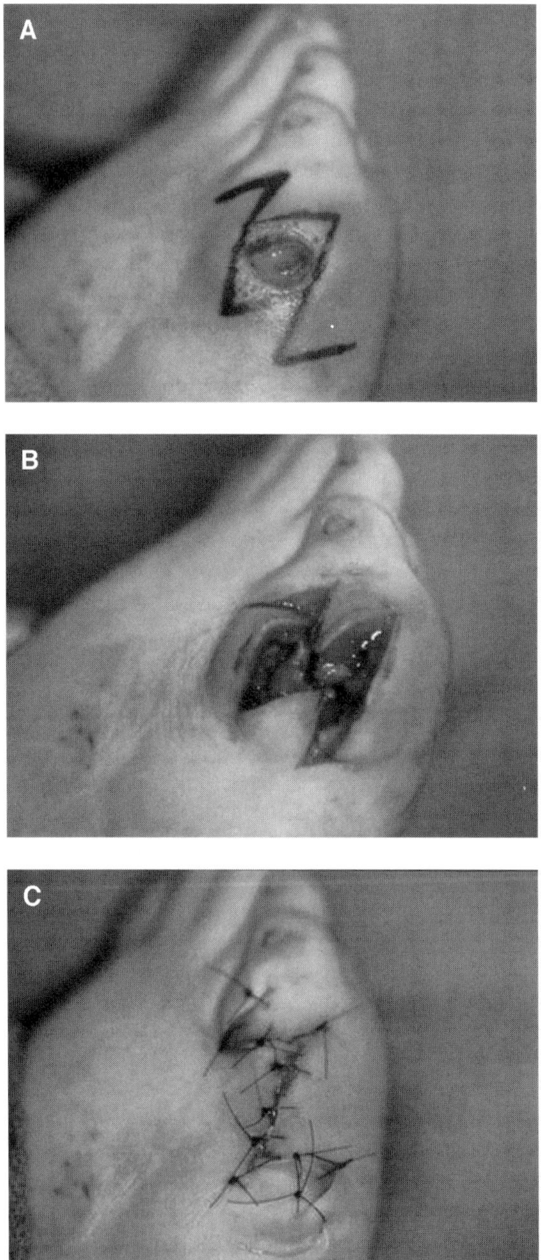

Fig. 8. Double-Z rhomboid. (*A*) Flap planning. (*B*) Mobilization of the flaps. (*C*) Reciprocal transposition of the flaps and closure. (*D*) Appearance after 4 months.

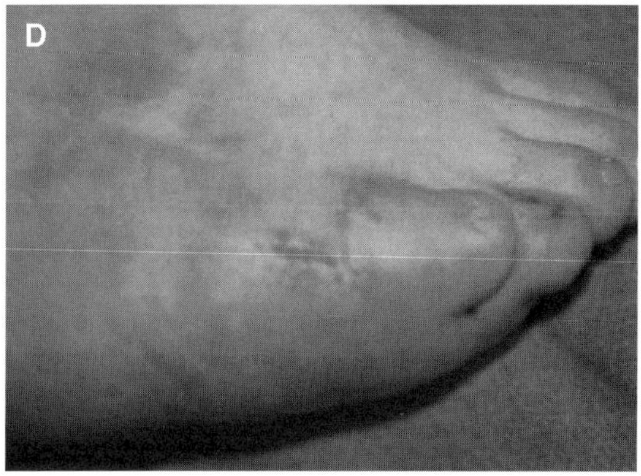

Fig. 8 (*continued*).

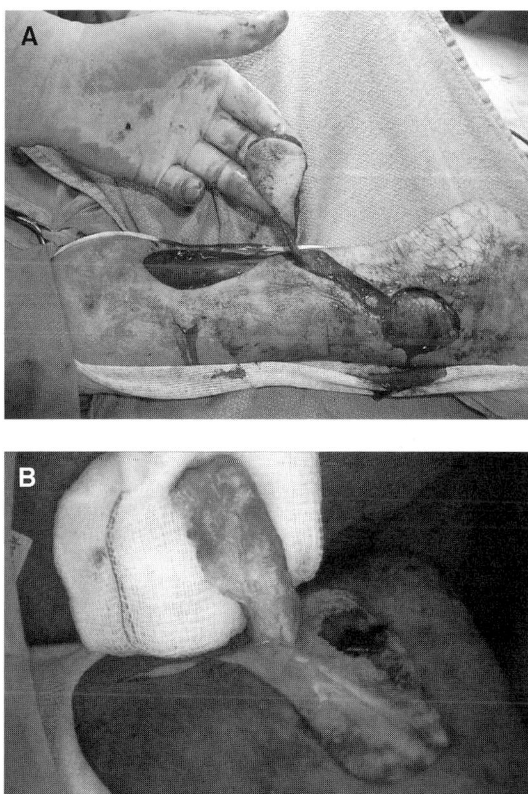

Fig. 9. Types of pedicle flaps. (*A*) An island flap supplied by a pedicle based on the sural artery. (*B*) A peninsula flap based on the lateral calcaneal artery.

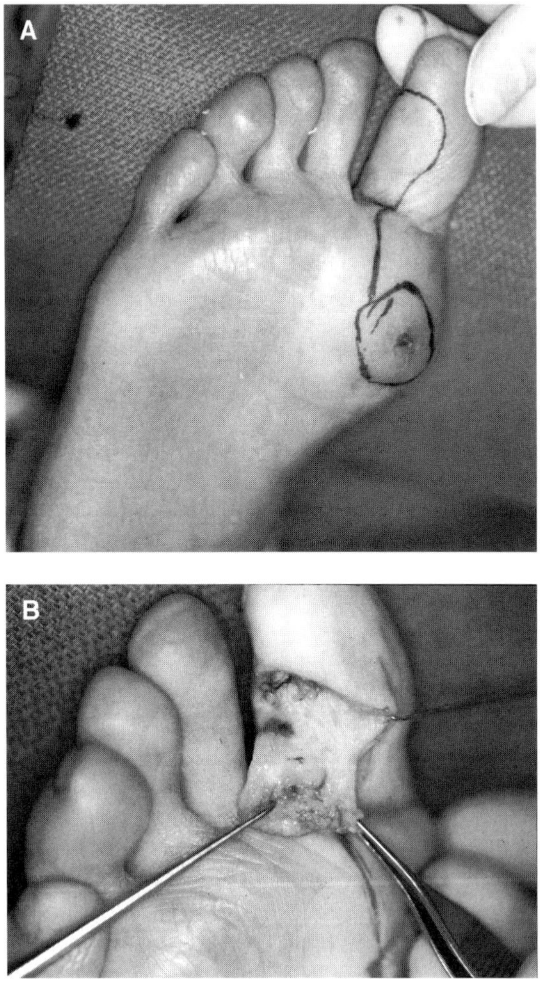

Fig. 10. A digital artery flap. (*A*) Flap planning. An island of skin and subcutaneous tissue from the great toe. (*B*) The flap is raised at the periosteum, and the digital vessels are visible. (*C*) The island flap is reversed and inset into the defect. A skin graft has been used to cover the donor site.

It has been said that the next best skin for closure of a defect is best next skin. Adjacent tissue has the characteristics of all of the adjacent tissues and typically may provide a viable coverage option. These flaps can be completed in a single stage or may be delayed, depending upon the host and the nature of the wound at the time of reconstruction. Infection must be appropriately addressed and controlled before any consideration is given to coverage of these defects. It is para-

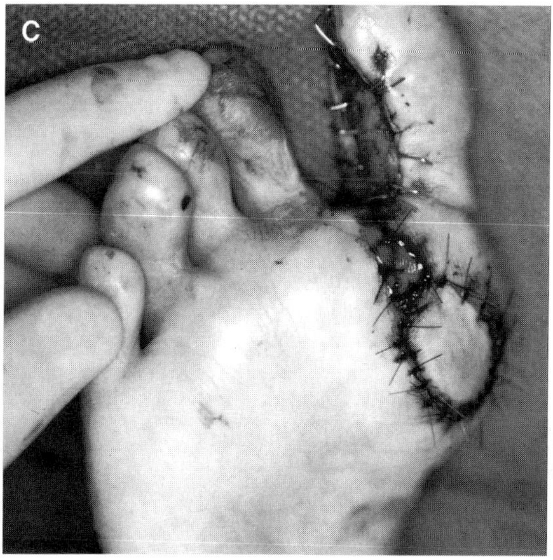

Fig. 10 (*continued*).

mount that these patients and their wounds are appropriately analyzed for perfusion and wound-healing potentials before considering a local flap reconstruction [28].

Pedicle flaps

Pedicle flaps are defined as areas of tissue that have a well-identifiable neurovascular supply that is expected to remain patent if that area of tissue is moved. Pedicle flaps may be in the form of an island, where the skin is circumscribed, or as a peninsula in which case the skin is continuous (Fig. 9). The development of flaps that are based on a specific neurovascular axis or stalk has greatly improved the reconstructive surgeon's ability to repair defects in the foot.

Pedicle flaps may be raised from tissue immediately adjacent to a soft tissue defect or from a site at a distance from the defect. A particular advantage of pedicle flaps over local flaps is that they are harvested from areas that are not weight-bearing, so that if the flap should fail, the original defect does not become larger as a result of that failure. Pedicle flaps may be of various tissues types, including fasciocutaneous, adipofascial, and muscular. Each tissue composite has specific indications in the foot and ankle. Because the foot and lower leg normally have a rich collateral network of vessels, pedicle flaps may be developed with an antegrade blood flow or with a retrograde flow. Retrograde flow is where the normal flow in the arteries and veins are reversed as a result of a pressure gradient. This permits the development of a flap that can be raised from a proximal donor site on the foot or lower leg and moved to a more distal location.

Digital artery island flaps

Replacement of soft tissue defects on the hand by neurocutaneous islands, taken from the sides of the fingers, was described by Littler, Atasoy, and others [29–33]. The successes from these operations eventually led to similar flaps being developed from the toes and used to cover defects on the foot [34,35]. A flap may be raised from either side of any toe, and its pedicle is based on the digital artery, vein, and nerve. Typically, the lateral surface of the great toe and the medial surface of the fifth toe are used more commonly because the metatarsal arteries from which they arise are inherently the longest and provide easiest dissection and a greater arc of rotation (Fig 10) [21]. These flaps are adipofascial, and once inset are able to move with the surrounding tissue during weight-bearing activities. These flaps are commonly used to cover defects on the ball of the foot, although with careful dissection, the metatarsal artery may be skeletonized from the plantar arch to provide coverage as far proximally as the heel and ankle [36].

Instep flaps (medial plantar artery flaps)

The arch of the foot was identified as an excellent source of replacement tissue for either the ball of the foot or the heel, because of the similarity in tissue properties. Flaps raised from the instep are supplied by two separate angiosomes, the collateral flow from the dorsalis pedis and cutaneous perforators from the medial plantar artery. When these flaps are developed as medially based peninsulas, both blood supplies are preserved. However, in the presence of a healthy plantar arterial arch, the flap may be converted to an island, based only on the medial plantar artery. The medial plantar artery may then be transected so that the island may be mobilized on its vascular pedicle. This greatly increases the effective arc of rotation of the flap. These flaps may be raised with either antegrade or retrograde flow [37–41]. If the flaps are distally based (retrograde), they can be used to resurface the forefoot (Fig 11A), whereas a proximally based pedicle will allow for rotation proximally to close defects of the heel (Fig. 11B).

Reverse flow sural artery neurofasciocutaneous flaps

These flaps are useful in covering defects on the ankle, lower leg, and heel, areas that historically have been difficult to cover. Fasciocutaneous islands of tissue can be raised from the posterolateral surface of the leg and are based on the arteries that accompany the median branch of the sural nerve, the arterial commitantes of the lesser saphenous vein. These vessels anastomose with a series of septocutaneous perforators from the peroneal artery. The most distal perforator, and subsequently the most distal pivot point for any flap designed on this pedicle, is usually found approximately 5 cm proximal to the lateral malleolus. The donor site may be closed primarily or with a skin graft, depending on the size of the flap (Fig. 12).

The distally based sural artery flap was first described in the early 1980s and gained popularity in the early 1990s [42–46]. Wounds of the lower leg, ankle, and heel have been notoriously difficult areas to cover, often requiring free muscle

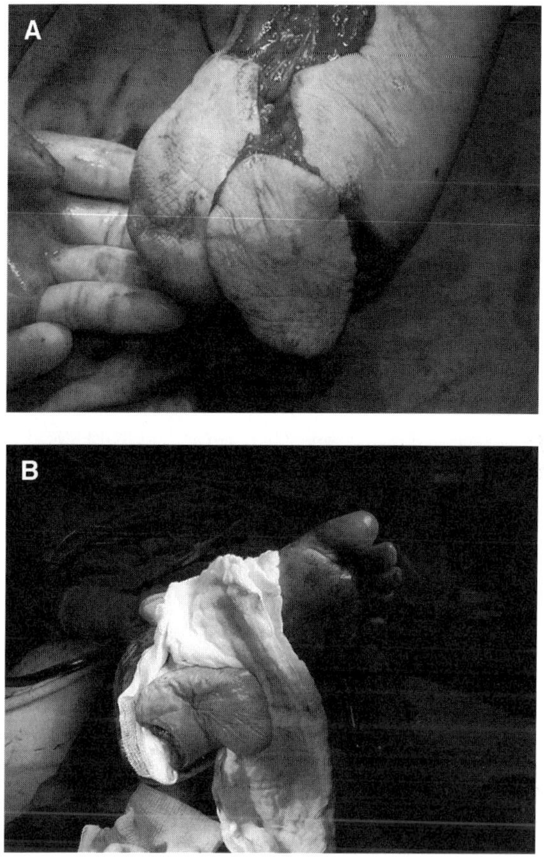

Fig. 11. (*A*) A retrograde flap based on the medial plantar artery and several cutaneous perforators. The flap was used to cover a large forefoot defect. (*B*) An antegrade flap based on the medial plantar artery and cutaneous perforators. It was raised from the instep and moved proximally to cover a large plantar heel defect.

flaps. With the advent of reverse flow flaps, including those of similar design based on the saphenous nerve, the superficial peroneal nerve and the supramaleollar flap, have all but rendered free muscle flaps irrelevant.

Muscle flaps

Muscles have been used to provide bulk to a defect and provide well-vascularized coverage to exposed bone. They may be developed as free flaps or as local pedicled flaps. Muscles have been classified on their pattern of vascular supply [47,48]. Type II muscles, which have a major pedicle and several minor ones, are generally used for this purpose. The muscle may be mobilized by releasing the origin and insertion as well as sacrificing the minor pedicles while preserving the major pedicle to perfuse the entire muscle. Type II muscles in the

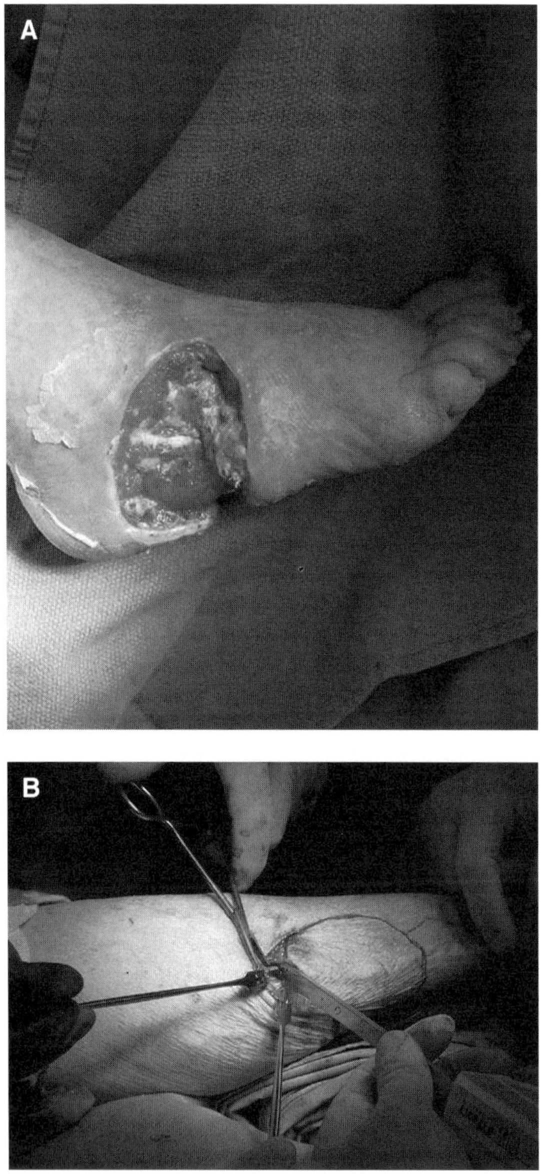

Fig. 12. Sural artery flap. (*A*) A large plantar-lateral hindfoot defect with exposed peroneal tendons and calcaneocuboid joint. (*B*) Elevation of the fasciocutaneous island from the back of the leg. (*C*) Mobilization of the pedicle. (*D*) Appearance of the flap at 4 months. The donor site was skin grafted.

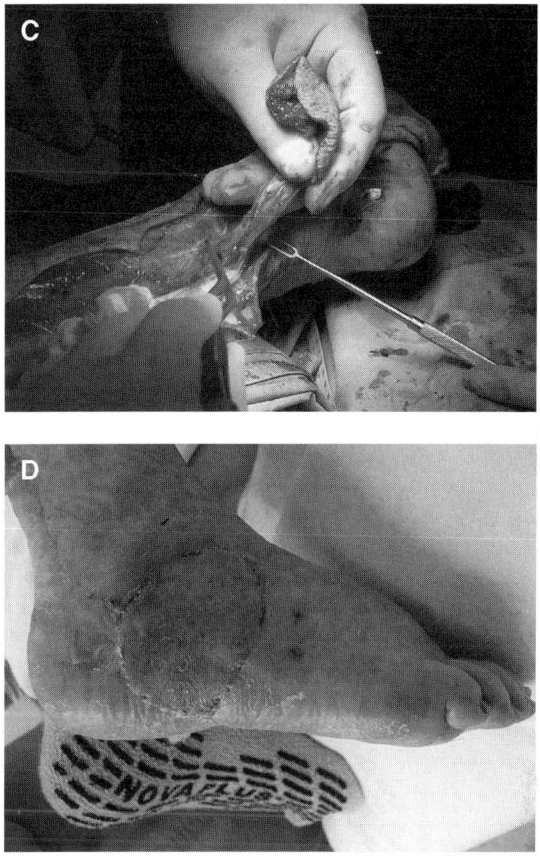

Fig. 12 (*continued*).

foot include the abductor hallucis, the abductor digiti minimi, the flexor digitorum brevis, and the extensor digitorum brevis. These muscles tend to be atrophic as a result of neuropathy in the patient who has diabetes, and so care should be taken to avoid overestimating the size of these muscles. Once the muscles are sutured to the recipient dermis and fascia, the muscle may be covered with a split-thickness skin graft. The skin graft is then protected with a stent dressing to prevent the skin graft from dislodging.

Extensor digitorum brevis

The blood supply to this muscle is based primarily on the lateral tarsal artery. It may be mobilized on this vessel to cover defects in the lateral tarsus, including the sinus tarsi (Fig. 13).

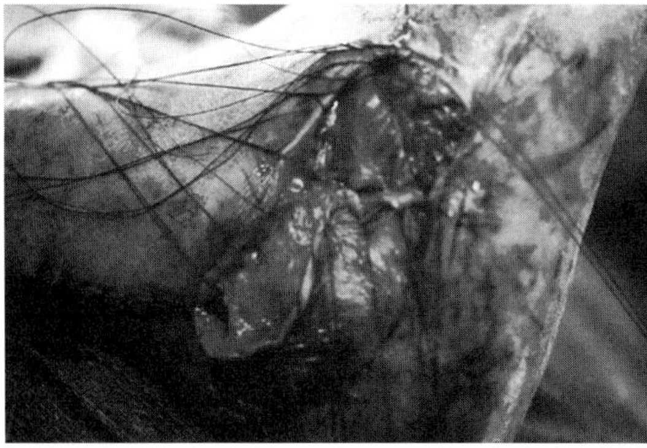

Fig. 13. Extensor digitorum brevis flap. The muscle was turned over on itself to cover the peroneal tendons. It was covered with a skin graft.

Abductor hallucis

The abductor hallucis's major pedicle is proximal so that its arc of rotation will allow it to be used along the medial edge of the foot, up to the medial malleolus (Fig. 14).

Flexor digitorum brevis

The flexor digitorum brevis is a muscle of significant bulk, which receives two major pedicles, one each from the medial plantar artery and the lateral plantar artery. Its attachment to the tendon slips may be severed and the muscle may be turned over on itself to cover defects of the midfoot and heel (Fig. 15).

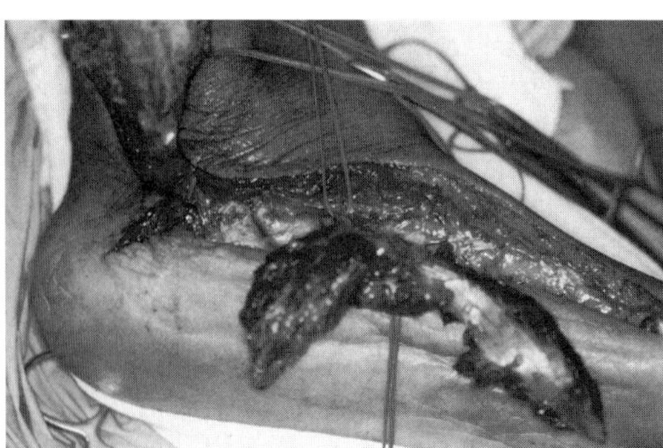

Fig. 14. Abductor hallucis muscle flap.

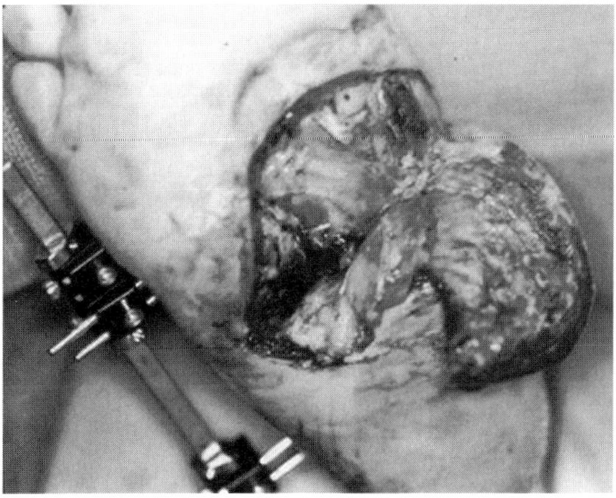

Fig. 15. Flexor digitorum brevis flap. This flap was mobilized and placed against an intercalary autogenous tricortical graft to enhance vascularization of the grafted tissue. This was done as part of a lateral column stabilization and soft tissue reconstruction.

Abductor digiti minimi

This is the smallest of the intrinsic foot muscles that are used for coverage. The muscle's origin is the lateral tubercle of the calcaneus and it inserts into the fifth metatarsal styloid. It is the smallest of the intrinsic muscles, but can aid in providing coverage of the lateral aspect of the calcaneal tuber (Fig. 16).

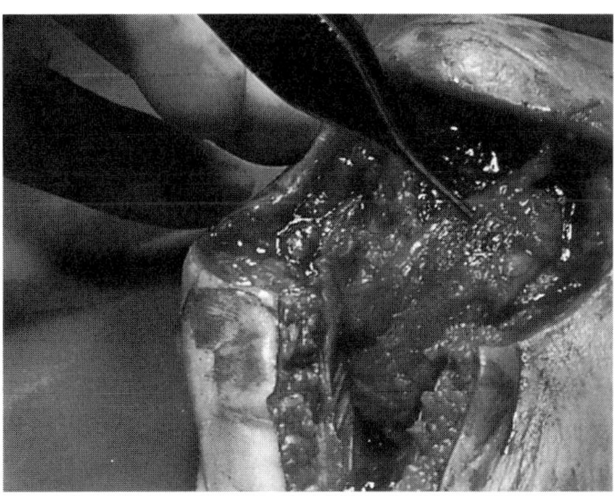

Fig. 16. Abductor digiti minimi flap. This flap was raised to provide coverage to a lateral heel defect. It was covered with a skin graft.

Summary

Treatment of wounds in the diabetic foot presents a set of difficult problems that requires "out of the box" thinking. The traditional approach of off-loading these wounds is often expensive, time-consuming, and in some cases seemingly never ending. The literature speaks loudly for a change in the philosophy of treating chronic wounds. When developing a team to treat chronic diabetic wounds, a reconstructive foot and ankle surgeon trained in these techniques is an appropriate addition to the team.

References

[1] Saraffian SK. Anatomy of the foot and ankle. In: Saraffian SK, editor. Functional anatomy of the foot & ankle. 2nd edition. Philadelphia: J.B. Lippincott; 1993. p. 346–8.
[2] Connoly JE, Wrobel JS, Anderson RF. Primary closure of infected diabetic foot wounds. A report of closed instillation in 30 cases. J Am Podiatr Med Assoc 2000;90:175–82.
[3] Tennvall GR, Apelqvist J, Eneroth M. Costs of deep foot infections in patients with diabetes mellitus. Pharmacoeconomics 2000;18:225–38.
[4] Apelqvist J, Ragnarson-Tennvall G, Persson U, Larsson J. Diabetic foot ulcers in a multidisciplinary setting. An economic analysis of primary healing and healing with amputation. J Intern Med 1994;235:463–71.
[5] Reiffel RS, McCarthy JG. Coverage of heel and sole defects: a new subfacsial arterialized flap. Plast Reconstr Surg 1980;66:250–60.
[6] Colen LB, Replogle SL, Mathes SJ. The V-Y plantar flap for reconstruction of the forefoot. Plast Reconstr Surg 1988;81:220–7.
[7] May JW, Rohrich RJ. Foot reconstruction using free microvascular muscle flaps with skin grafts. Clin Plast Surg 1986;13:681–9.
[8] Dockery GL, Christensen JC. Principles and descriptions of designed skin flaps for use on the lower extremity. Clin Podiatr Med Surg 1986;3:563–77.
[9] Converse JM, Uhlschmid GK, Ballantyne DL. Plasmatic circulation of skin grafts. Plast Reconstr Surg 1969;43:495–9.
[10] Converse JM, Smahel J, Ballantyne DL, et al. Inosculation of vessels of skin graft and host bed: a fortuitous encounter. Br J Plast Surg 1975;28:274–82.
[11] Smahel J. The healing of skin grafts. Clin Plast Surg 1977;4:409–24.
[12] Donato MC, Novicki DC, Blume PA. Skin grafting: historic and practical approaches. Clin Podiatr Med Surg 2000;17:561–98.
[13] Frangos SG, Kilaru S, Blume PA, et al. Classification of diabetic foot ulcers. improving communication. Int J Angiol 2002;11:1–7.
[14] Knox RC, Dutch W, Blume PA, Sumpio BE. Diabetic foot disease. Int J Angiol 2000;9:1–6.
[15] Sumpio BE, Blume PA. Contemporary management of foot ulcers, trends in vascular surgery. In: Pierce WH, Matsumura JS, Yao JST, editors. Chicago: Precept Press; 2002. p. 277–90.
[16] Attinger CE, Bulan E, Blume PA. Surgical debridement. The key to successful wound healing and reconstruction. Clin Podiatr Med Surg 2000;17:599–630.
[17] Blume PA, Paragas LK, Sumpio BE, Attinger CE. Single-stage surgical treatment of noninfected diabetic foot ulcers. J Plast Reconstr Surg 2002;109:601–9.
[18] Paragas L, Attinger C, Blume PA. Local flaps. Clin Podiatr Med Surg 2000;17:267–318.
[19] Hidalgo DA, Shaw WW. Anatomic basis of plantar flap design. Plast Reconstr Surg 1986;78: 627–36.
[20] Attinger CE. Use of soft tissue techniques for salvage of the diabetic foot. In: Kominski SJ, editor. Medical and surgical management of the diabetic foot. St. Louis, MO: Mosby Year Book Inc.; 1994. p. 323–66.

[21] Attinger C, Cooper P, Blume P. Vascular anatomy of the foot and ankle. Operative Techniques in Plastic & Reconstructive Surgery 1997;4:183–98.
[22] Attinger C. Soft tissue coverage for lower extremity trauma. Orthop Clin North Am 1995;26: 295–334.
[23] Zimany A. The bi-lobed flap. Plast Reconstr Surg 1953;11:424–34.
[24] Limberg AA. Mathematical principles of local plastic procedures on the surface of the human body. Leningrad: Medgriz; 1946.
[25] Limberg AA. Design of local flaps. In: Gibson T, editor. Modern trends in plastic surgery. 2nd edition. London: Butterworths; 1966. p. 38–61.
[26] Ashbell TS. The rhomboid excision and Limberg flap reconstruction in difficult tense skin areas. Plast Reconstr Surg 1982;4:724.
[27] Cuono CB. Double Z plasty repair of large and small rhombic defects: the double Z rhomboid. Plast Reconstr Surg 1983;71:658–66.
[28] Blume PA, Dey HM, Daley LJ, et al. Diagnosis of pedal osteomyelitis with Tc-99-M HMPAO labeled leukocytes. J Foot Ankle Sug 1997;36:120–6.
[29] Littler JW. The neurovascular pedicle method of digital transposition for reconstruction of the thumb. Plast Reconstr Surg 1953;12:303–19.
[30] Littler JW. Neurovascular pedicle transfer of tissue in reconstructive surgery of the hand. J Bone Joint Surg 1956;38:917.
[31] Atasoy E, Iokimides E, Kasden ML, et al. Reconstruction of the amputated finger tip with a triangular volar flap. J Bone Joint Surg 1970;52:921–6.
[32] Snow JW. The use of a volar flap for the repair of finger tip amputations: a preliminary report. Plast Reconstr Surg 1967;40:163–8.
[33] Moberg E. Aspects of sensation in reconstructive surgery of the extremity. J Bone Joint Surg 1964;46:817.
[34] Buncke HJ, Colen LB. An island flap from the first web space of the foot to cover plantar ulcers. Br J Plast Sur 1980;33:242–4.
[35] Colen LB, Buncke HJ. Neurovascular island flaps from the plantar vessels and nerves for foot reconstruction. Ann Plast Surg 1984;12:327–32.
[36] Morain WD. Island toe flaps in neurotrophic ulcers of the foot and ankle. Ann Plast Surg 1984; 13:1–8.
[37] Bhandari PS, Sobti C. Reverse flow instep island flap. Plast Reconstr Surg 1999;103:1986–9.
[38] Narsette T. Anatomic design of a sensate plantar flap. Ann Plast Surg 1997;38:538–9.
[39] Miyamoto Y, Ikuta Y, Shigeti S, Yamura M. Current concepts of instep island flap. Ann Plast Surg 1987;19:97–102.
[40] Butler CE, Chevray P. Retrograde flow medial plantar island flap reconstruction of distal forefoot, toe and web space defects. Ann Plast Surg 2002;49:196–201.
[41] Baker GL, Newton D, Franklin JD. Fasciocutaneous island flap based on the medial plantar artery: clinical applications for leg, ankle and forefoot. Plast Reconstr Surg 1990;85:47–58.
[42] Donski PK, Fogdestam I. Distally based fasciocutaneous flap from the sural region: a preliminary report. Scand J Reconstr Surg 1983;17:191–6.
[43] Hasegawa M, Torii S, Katoh H, Esaki S. The distally based superficial sural artery flap. Plast Reconstr Surg 1994;93:1012–20.
[44] Jeng SF, Wei FC. Distally based sural island flap for foot and ankle reconstruction. Plast Reconstr Surg 1997;99:744–50.
[45] Huisinga RL, Houpt P, Dijkstra R, et al. The distally based sural artery flap. Ann Plast Surg 1998; 41:58–65.
[46] Jeng SF, Wei FC, Kuo YR. Salvage of the distal foot using the distally based sural island flap. Ann Plast Surg 1999;43:499–505.
[47] Geddles CR, Morris SF, Neligan PC. Perforator flaps: evolution, classification, and applications. Ann Plast Surg 2003;50:90–9.
[48] Attinger CE, Ducic I, Zelen C. The use of local muscle flaps in foot and ankle reconstruction. Clin Podiatr Med Surg 2000;17:681–711.

Clin Podiatr Med Surg
20 (2003) 783–792

CLINICS IN
PODIATRIC
MEDICINE AND
SURGERY

Elective surgery of the diabetic foot

Lee R. Sayner, DPM, Barry I. Rosenblum, DPM*,
John M. Giurini, DPM

*Department of Surgery, Harvard Medical School, Division of Podiatry,
Beth Israel Deaconess Medical Center, One Deaconess Road, Boston, MA 02215, USA*

The diabetic foot has always been a challenge to health care practitioners. Historically, surgical management in this area was primarily limited to treatment of ulceration and acute infection. Many surgeons had reservations about operating on patients who had diabetes, perhaps because of fear of poor outcomes or because of a patient's medical comorbidities, such as peripheral vascular disease. Surgical management was avoided before the development of ulceration or infection and was only considered as a reaction to an already established problem. More practitioners now appreciate the role that elective diabetic surgery has in the treatment and prevention of ulceration, infection, and amputation [1]. Prophylactic surgery can be a definitive treatment when conservative therapy has failed to prevent or heal ulceration, when ulcerations are stabilized but prone to further breakdown, or when ulcers recur with or without the presence of osteomyelitis [2,3]. In addition to limb salvage or avoidance of ablative types of procedures, such as debridement and amputation, surgery can be reconstructive, allowing for stabilization once a foot has been impacted by neuropathy and its sequelae [4].

It is widely acknowledged that foot ulceration with associated infection is one of the leading causes of hospitalization for patients who have diabetes. The sociologic and economic costs of hospitalizations and amputations are significant [5]. The goal of performing surgery when foot abnormalities are in their early stages is to avoid more destructive and debilitating ablative surgery later.

Risk factors for ulceration and amputations

The pathophysiology of diabetic foot ulceration needs to be understood fully if such conditions are to be treated successfully. The most significant predisposing factor for the development of ulcerations is peripheral sensory polyneuropathy.

* Corresponding author.
E-mail address: brosenbl@caregroup.harvard.edu (B.I. Rosenblum).

doi:10.1016/S0891-8422(03)00073-9

Loss of protective sensation leads to an inability to perceive the pain of micro- and macrotrauma to the foot. Irritation from shoe gear, wounds from foreign objects, or elevated pressures from faulty biomechanics often go unnoticed. Increased focal plantar foot pressures have been shown to frequently lead to ulceration [6]. Diabetics often suffer from autonomic neuropathy, manifesting as a dysfunction of the sympathetic nervous system; absence of sweat production and loss of skin temperature regulation leads to dry, stiff, scaly skin with cracks and fissures. Perfusion abnormalities secondary to autonomic neuropathy may predispose the patient to Charcot deformity. Motor neuropathy is also seen in diabetics, with weakness of intrinsic musculature predisposing to pedal deformities. Intrinsic muscle wasting leads to progressive deformities, such as hammertoes and plantarflexed metatarsals, and contributes to areas of high focal pressure. Motor neuropathy can exacerbate preexisting ankle equinus deformity, which places greater stress beneath the forefoot during ambulation [7,8].

Peripheral vascular disease (PVD) is commonly seen in the diabetic population, although it is rarely a primary risk factor for ulceration [16]. Once an ulcer has occurred, however, the presence of PVD can prevent healing and slow the resolution of infection. A thorough vascular exam should be performed on all patients who have diabetes. If noninvasive vascular studies reveal the presence of poor circulation, consultation with a vascular surgeon is indicated. Though it is sometimes necessary to urgently operate on a diabetic foot (ie, with incision and drainage of an abscess), truly elective surgeries should wait until revascularization procedures restore blood flow necessary for healing.

Goals of surgery

Prophylactic surgery on the diabetic foot is generally performed with the goal of preventing more advanced and debilitating conditions from developing. The specific aim, however, is to reduce the risk of foot ulceration and amputation by correcting structural deformities leading to cutaneous compromise. Patients with lesions who have a history of minor infection and have reconstructible deformity often do well with elective surgery. Eliminating focal areas of increased pressure, primarily over bony prominences, and providing a stable plantigrade foot for ambulation, are methods of preventing recurrent ulceration and debilitating consequences [3,9]. Elective surgery is also indicated when Charcot neuroarthropathic changes or previous ablative procedures have resulted in ulcer-prone high-risk extremities. Other goals include creating a foot that can be successfully accommodated in custom shoes, an ankle foot orthosis (AFO), or braces.

Preoperative evaluation

Proper timing of procedures is as important as the selection of the type of procedure. Before correction of any underlying deformity, any acute infection should be converted to a chronic infection or a clean colonized wound. Abscesses need to be drained, and any necrotic or infected tissue or bone should be sharply excised at this time. More definitive reconstructive procedures are performed once a clean, uninfected wound has been created [5].

A multidisciplinary team approach yields the best result. Consultation with services such as medicine, vascular surgery, plastic surgery, endocrinology, and nutrition is frequently helpful. If there is a concern about the vascular supply to the foot, a vascular surgery consult can be obtained to better evaluate the arterial supply in the involved extremity. Initially, noninvasive testing may be necessary to assess perfusion. If there is still concern, arteriography may be indicated as a possible prelude to arterial reconstruction. Reconstructive procedures following revascularization have been shown to improve the limb salvage rate [10]. The expertise of an endocrinologist is helpful in managing hyperglycemia, as elevated blood glucose levels may have deleterious effects on the immune system, such as delayed wound closure, defects in chemotaxis and granulocyte activity, collagen synthesis, and erythrocyte function [11]. Larger skin defects or difficult wounds may require plastic surgery for advanced flaps or grafting.

Patient selection is especially important. Noncompliance can have disastrous results. Often, the length of immobilization or non–weight-bearing in the patient who has neuropathy is extended longer than in patients with normal sensation. It is often predictable that patients with peripheral sensory neuropathy will be fully weight-bearing despite instructions that allow for only partial weight-bearing. The lack of pain sensation does not allow for feedback to the patient that they are bearing excessive weight in the same way it would in patients with normal pain sensation [5]. Patients with active Charcot neuroarthropathy should wait until the process reaches the coalescent phase before undergoing elective procedures [12]. Elective diabetic foot surgery should not be performed on limbs with inadequate vascularity to heal an incision. There are some who recommend avoiding elective clean surgery when infected tissue is being debrided [13].

Surgical procedures

Nails and lesser digits

Chronic recurrent ingrown nails are a common condition in patients who have diabetes. Acutely infected nail borders are treated with partial nail avulsion, whereas recurrent conditions are addressed with nail border matrixectomy. The commonly performed phenol and alcohol procedure can be safely performed in patients with adequate pedal perfusion [9]. It is important that the patient have enough circulation to heal the wound and combat infection. The prolonged drainage sometimes seen afterward may be prevented instead by performing sharp excisional matrixectomy in patients with marginal perfusion.

Hammer toe deformities in the patient who has neuropathy frequently develop ulceration because of the pressure from shoe gear or bony prominences. Simple digital procedures, if performed early, may prevent later amputation. Attempts should be made to salvage the second toe, in particular, to avoid the development or worsening of a hallux abducto valgus deformity. Selection of an appropriate digital procedure depends on the reducibility of the contracture, the location of ulceration, and the extent of infection.

Flexible hammer toes may be addressed with a simple percutaneous flexor tenotomy procedure, with any superficial distal ulcers left to heal by secondary intention. When osteomyelitis of the distal phalanx is also present, the flexor tenotomy may be performed in conjunction with phalangeal resection and ulcer excision. The wound may be closed primarily or packed open if residual infection is suspected. When soft tissue involvement is extensive, a terminal Syme's procedure may be warranted.

For semirigid or rigid hammer toes, arthroplasty or arthrodesis of the proximal interphalangeal joint are performed. Converging semielliptical incisions facilitate full-thickness removal of ulcerations. One must ensure that adequate resection of infected bone has been performed. In areas of active infection, internal fixation is to be avoided.

First ray

The first ray is a common area for ulceration to occur in the patient who has diabetic neuropathy. Ulceration of the hallux or first metatarsal head region are not uncommon. It has been well-documented that there is an increased risk of transfer lesion, infection, and possible amputation once the first ray has been lost. Other complications may occur secondary to loss of the great toe or first ray. The increased pronatory forces experienced by the remaining forefoot may lead to stress fractures of the lesser metatarsals, and possibly Charcot collapse of the more proximal medial column.

Hallux interphalangeal joint arthroplasty is warranted when conservative treatment fails to maintain healing of ulcers of the great toe [14]. Ulcerations involving the hallux are fairly common and may be secondary to abnormal first ray biomechanics, such as excessive pronation or hallux limitus [15]. In cases of faulty foot function at the first metatarsophalangeal joint, procedures designed to improve function of that joint may be indicated, such as Keller arthroplasty or cheilectomy. Enlarged bony prominences or interphalangeal sesamoid bones may also cause lesions.

The hallux arthroplasty is usually performed through a dorsal approach. Various other incision types, such as serpentine, longitudinal, and transverse have been used. Plantar incisions may be considered if there is an ulcer to be excised. The head of the proximal phalanx is resected, along with any interphalangeal sesamoids, following capsulotomy and transection of the collateral ligaments. The resulting toe is rectus, with little or no instability at the interphalangeal level. A pseudarthrosis or fibrous union develops.

Hallux interphalangeal joint fusion may be indicated for instability of this area, or for distal tip ulcerations caused by rigid hallux hammer toe deformity.

Surgical approach is similar to that for arthroplasty, but the cartilage on the base of the distal phalanx is also resected. Various methods of fixation have proved successful, including Kirschner wires, monofilament wires, or cancellous screw. Prolonged periods of postoperative non–weight-bearing, perhaps 6 to 8 weeks, are necessary for fusion to occur, making arthroplasty without fixation a more appealing procedure.

Keller or Keller-Mayo arthroplasty procedures can address chronic recurring ulcerations of the first ray, osteoarthritis of the first metatarsophalangeal joint, and hallux rigidus [16]. The Keller arthroplasty may be performed from a dorsal approach, with a plantar ulcer left to heal by secondary intention. The prevention of amputation or recurrence of ulceration can necessitate these joint-destructive surgeries. Possible complications of the Keller procedure include lack of hallux purchase, dorsal toe contracture, transfer ulcers, or lesser metatarsal stress fractures.

If a plantar wound directly involves the first metatarsophalangeal joint, however, the authors recommend joint resection through a plantar approach with ulcer excision; converging semielliptical incisions are made to excise the ulceration completely. The incisions must be long enough to avoid tension when the wound is closed, and the flexor hallucis longus tendon and both sesamoids often must be sacrificed to avoid residual focus of infection. The base of the proximal phalanx, especially the plantar condyle, should be resected if there are any clinical signs of osteomyelitis. The articular surface of the first metatarsal head is resected to remove potential sources of bone and joint infection, to provide a healthy vascular bed to support granulation tissue, and to allow delivery of antibiotics to the site through the exposed bleeding cancellous surface. The metatarsal head must be resected at an angle that minimizes plantar bony spicules.

Sesamoidectomy can be performed for ulcerations plantar to the first metatarsal head. If there is no evidence of osteomyelitis of the metatarsal and no significant degenerative change noted within the joint, then one or both sesamoids may be excised to decrease plantar first ray pressure [17]. The long flexor tendon should usually be protected, but may need excision if ulceration is contiguous with the tendon. Repair of the tendon may be indicated if there is damage noted at the time of operation.

Sesamoidectomy may alter the first ray biomechanics but may result in complete ulcer resolution with the advantage of an earlier return to weight-bearing status. Where there is a rigidly plantarflexed first ray, a first metatarsal dorsiflexory osteotomy or first metatarsal-medial cuneiform fusion should be considered instead of removing the sesamoids [4]. Isolated tibial sesamoidectomy through a medial incision is usually sufficient for patients with mild hallux valgus deformity. If there exists the likelihood of worsening of this deformity, then a first metatarsal osteotomy should be considered. For the rectus or pes cavus foot types, both sesamoids may need excision; the surgeon must be aware that this may predispose the patient to a hallux hammer toe. If this condition already exists, a hallux interphalangeal fusion could be considered as an adjunct procedure.

Lesser metatarsals

Lesions located plantar to the lesser metatarsal heads develop as a result of excessive focal pressure secondary to plantarflexed metatarsals, limited joint mobility, digital contracture, or transfer lesions from previous surgeries [18–20]. Procedural selection is dependent on the extent of ulceration and whether osteomyelitis is present. Lesser metatarsal osteotomy may be considered for treatment of ulcerations that do not involve bone or joint. The approach is usually dorsal, and the metatarsal is dorsiflexed or elevated to alleviate plantar pressure. Fixation may be used if there is no cellulitis. Without the use of fixation, postoperative non–weight-bearing is recommended for 6 to 8 weeks. Complications of lesser metatarsal osteotomies include transfer calluses or ulcerations. Delayed union or nonunion is usually asymptomatic. To prevent transfer lesions, osteotomy of multiple metatarsals may be considred.

A resection of a lesser metatarsal head will more likely lead to plantar ulcer resolution but will also be more likely to result in a transfer lesion. The presence of osteomyelitis, however, may leave the surgeon with little choice. Some prefer resection through a clean dorsal incision and allowing the ulcer to heal by secondary intention; others advocate a plantar approach with complete excision of infected tissue followed by primary closure. Regardless of the approach, consideration must be given to closure at the time of the procedure. If the wound created is sufficiently large enough so as to not allow for a tension-free closure, then a local flap may be considered. Depending on the extent of infection and the presence of osteomyeltits, closure may be done as a single-stage procedure or a delayed method [21].

The base of the proximal phalanx must also be inspected for signs of osteomyelitis, with appropriate resection performed. Accommodative orthotics may help distribute forefoot pressures more evenly following the procedure. Possible complications include wound dehiscence, transfer lesions, stress fractures, and short or flail toes. With isolated metatarsal head resections, the associated toe can often contract, shorten, and assume a more dorsal location; this creates an uneven metatarsal parabola, and the stress upon the adjacent metatarsals may lead to Charcot neuroarthropathy in that area [22]. This procedure, however, is preferred to resection of the ray (toe and metatarsal head) [23].mbf

Multiple metatarsal head procedures are often necessary in diabetics as a result of transfer ulceration or osteomyelitis. If more than one metatarsal head has been resected, or needs to be resected, a panmetatarsal head resection is often indicated. The selection of this procedure to definitively treat chronic ulcerations in the neuropathic foot was originally described by Jacobs [24]. Over time, it has replaced the transmetatarsal amputation as the procedure of choice for patients with recurrent forefoot ulcerations following previous metatarsal head resection [24]. Multiple approaches have been used for this procedure. Most commonly, osteomyelitic metatarsal head and infected tissue is excised by way of a plantar approach and closed primarily; the other metatarsal heads are resected through dorsal incisions. Some surgeons prefer to excise bone from an incision site removed from an ulcer to minimize contamination of the underlying metatarsal;

some may also choose to pack the wound open and perform delayed primary closure [22,25,26].

Surgical resection of osteomyelitis may leave the surgeon with a large wound. These cases may require a local advancement or rotation flap to afford closure [21]. In addition, lesions of the forefoot that have failed to heal may have significant underlying ischemia. In these situations, vascular reconstruction may be necessary to allow for healing [10].

Midfoot procedures

In the diabetic population, elective midfoot procedures are usually performed for reconstruction of Charcot neuroarthropathic joint disease. The tarsometatarsal joints are usually involved, especially at the first metatarsal-medial cuneiform articulation. This condition can lead to disruption of joint architecture with collapse of the midfoot and resultant high focal plantar pressures with ulceration. When the midfoot retains osseous stability but there is a plantar prominence, a simple exostectomy may definitively resolve chronic ulceration [27]. If involved bone is not infected, the surgeon may perform the incision through adjacent healthy tissue; the osseous prominence is resected with power instrumentation or osteotome and then smoothed with a rasp or rongeur. When osteomyelitis is a concern, one may consider excising the ulcer and resecting the bone, followed by primary closure of the wound. The incision may need to be lengthened to allow for adequate skin reapproximation without excessive tension [27,28].

More severe Charcot joint processes can lead to extensive bone loss, joint dislocation, and midfoot instability. Simple exostectomy would not be appropriate, and a medial column fusion may be required to restore stability. When resecting the involved articular cartilage, removal of bone wedges may be necessary to achieve a plantigrade foot. Ulcers located centrally in the midfoot secondary to plantar cuboid subluxation may be particularly difficult to close primarily. Exostectomy with a fasciocutaneous flap may be required in these situations. Muscle flap can be used to decrease dead space following bone resection and to provide a layer of soft tissue between bone and skin. The flexor digitorum brevis is often used because of its location and ease of dissection; muscle is detached at its distal aspect and then laterally rotated [27,28]. Donor sites may be covered with split-thickness skin grafts

Rearfoot procedures

There are those situations where salvage procedures are required if a diabetic limb is to be saved from amputation. Heel ulcerations, for example, can result in prolonged disability; if ulceration progresses to the point of calcaneal osteomyelitis, many patients are then faced with the prospect of below-knee amputation. Partial or subtotal calcanectomy may be a viable option, however, with the goals of removing infected bone and soft tissue and ensuring that no plantar prominence remains. Ulcer excision with primary wound closure may be difficult to attain without rotational skin flaps or free flaps. Adequate perfusion to the heel is paramount to allow for healing. An ankle-foot orthosis is often required postoperatively.

When severe Charcot joint disease results in a flail hindfoot or ankle joint, the prognosis for the lower extremity is poor. Salvage procedures in this case may include primary fusion of involved joints to address the inherent instability and prevent chronic ulceration [22]. In some instances, talectomy with tibiocalcaneal fusion is indicated [29]. The heel should be fused in a neutral to slight valgus position.

When a significant rearfoot deformity has resulted in chronic nonhealing ulceration, reconstructive procedures may stabilize the foot and reduce areas of focal pressure. Rearfoot reconstructive surgery may include triple arthrodesis or ankle or pantalar joint fusion to restore function in the Charcot foot after the process has reached the coalescent phase. Joint resection with appropriate removal of bone wedges to restore a plantigrade foot, followed by arthrodesis of the involved joints, can reduce deformity and prevent significant disability. Bone graft may be required if there has been extensive bone resorption as a result of the neuroarthropathy. Electric bone stimulators can be a useful adjunct to promote union. Prolonged non–weight-bearing, perhaps for 3 to 4 months, may be necessary to achieve fusion.

Achilles tendon lengthening

The tendo-Achilles lengthening is a simple yet crucial component of many elective diabetic foot surgeries. Ankle joint equinus is prevalent in the pathologic diabetic foot, and may be exacerbated by intrinsic motor neuropathy. Lengthening of the Achilles tendon is often indicated in patients with partial foot amputations, forefoot deformities, or chronic ulcerations [7,30]. This procedure can be an important adjunct to surgical management of Charcot neuroarthropathy, as an uncompensated equinus deformity can initiate Charcot collapse. The tendon may be lengthened by way of a percutaneous release, a three-incision hemisection, or an open-slide lengthening in the frontal or sagittal plane. Regardless of the approach, an existing equinus deformity needs to be addressed.

Summary

It has been clearly demonstrated that elective surgery can be performed in the neuropathic foot. If infection is controlled and arterial supply is adequate, limb salvage can be greatly enhanced with an aggressive approach to elective procedures in the patient who has diabetes.

References

[1] Giurini JM, Rosenblum BI. The role of foot surgery in patients with diabetes. Clin Podiatr Med Surg 1995;12:119–27.
[2] Armstrong DG, Lavery LA, Stern S, Harkless LB. Is prophylactic diabetic foot surgery dangerous? J Foot Ankle Surg 1996;35(6):585–9.

[3] Frykberg RG, et al. Prophylactic surgery in the diabetic foot. In: Kominsky S, editor. Medical and surgical management of the diabetic foot. St. Louis (MO): Mosby; 1994. p. 394–438.
[4] Cooper PS. Orthopedic considerations in wound healing of the lower extremity. Foot Ankle Clin 2001;6:715–44.
[5] Giurini JM, Rosenblum BI. Surgical treatment of the diabetic foot. In: McGlamry ED, Banks AS, Downey MS, et al, editors. McGlamry's comprehensive textbook of foot and ankle surgery. 3rd edition. Baltimore: Lippincott Williams & Wilkins; 2001. p. 1595–616.
[6] Veves A, Murray HJ, Young MJ, et al. The risk of foot ulceration in diabetic patients with high foot pressures: a prospective study. Diabetologia 1992;35:660–8.
[7] Lin SS, Lee TH, Wapner KL. Plantar forefoot ulceration with equinus deformity of the ankle in diabetic patients: the effect of tendo-achilles lengthening and total contact casting. Orthopedics 1996;19:465–75.
[8] Niklas BJ. Prophylactic surgery in the diabetic foot. In: Frykberg RG, editor. The high risk foot in diabetes mellitus. New York: Churchill Livingstone; 1991. p. 513–41.
[9] Rosenblum BI, Pomposelli FB, Giurini JM, et al. Maximizing foot salvage by a combined approach to foot ischemia and neuropathic ulceration in patients with diabetes mellitus: a five year experience. Diabetes Care 1994;17:983–7.
[10] Pearl S, Khat I. Diabetes and healing: a review of the literature. J Foot Surg 1998;27:268–70.
[11] Papa J, Myerson M, Girard P. Salvage, with arthrodesis, in intractable diabetic neuropathic arthropathy of the foot and ankle. J Bone Joint Surg Am 1993;75:1056–66.
[12] Catanzariti AR. Prophylactic foot surgery in the diabetic patient. Adv Wound Care 1999;12(6): 312–7.
[13] Rosenblum BI, Giurini JM, Chrzan JS, et al. Preventing loss of the great toe with the hallux interphalangeal joint arthroplasty. J Foot Ankle Surg 1994;33:557–60.
[14] Dannels E. Neuropathic foot ulcer prevention in diabetic American Indians with hallux limitus. J Am Podiatr Med Assoc 1989;76:33–7.
[15] Downs DM, Jacobs RL. Treatment of resistant ulcers on the plantar surface of the great toe in diabetics. J Bone Joint Surg Am 1982;64:930–3.
[16] Giurini JM, Chrzan JS, Gibbons GW, et al. Sesamoidectomy for the treatment of chronic neuropathic ulcerations. J Am Podiatr Med Assoc 1991;81:167–73.
[17] Fernando DJ, Masson EA, Veves A, et al. Relationship of limited joint mobility to abnormal foot pressures and diabetic foot ulceration. Diabetes Care 1991;14:8–11.
[18] Tillo TH, Giurini JM, Habershaw GM, et al. Review of metatarsal osteotomies for the treatment of neuropathic ulcerations. J Am Podiatr Med Assoc 1990;80:211–7.
[19] Veves A, Sarnow MR, Giurini JM, et al. Differences in joint mobility and foot pressures between black and white diabetic patients. Diabet Med 1995;12:585–9.
[20] Blume PA, Paragas LK, Sumpio BE, Attinger CE. Single-stage surgical treatment of noninfected diabetic foot ulcers. Plast Reconstr Surg 2002;109:601–9.
[21] Banks AS. Elective diabetic foot surgery. In: McGlamry ED, Banks AS, Downey MS, editors. Comprehensive textbook of foot surgery. 2nd edition. Baltimore: Williams & Wilkins; 1992. p. 1371–83.
[22] Cohen M, Roman A, Malcolm WG. Panmetatarsal head resection and transmetatarsal amputation versus solitary partial ray resection in the neuropathic foot. J Foot Surg 1991;30:29–33.
[23] Giurini JM, Basile P, Chrzan JS, et al. Panmetatarsal head resection: a viable alternative to the transmetatarsal amputation. J Am Podiatr Med Assoc 1993;83:101–7.
[24] Jacobs RL. Hoffman procedure in the ulcerated diabetic neuropathic foot. Foot Ankle 1982;3: 142–9.
[25] Griffiths GD, Wieman TJ. Metatarsal head resection for diabetic foot ulcers. Arch Surg 1990; 125:264.
[26] Martin JD, Delbridge L, Reeve TS, et al. Radical treatment of mal perforans in diabetic patients with arterial insufficiency. J Vasc Surg 1990;12:264–8.
[27] Catanzariti AR, Mendicino R, Haverstock B. Ostectomy for diabetic neuroarthropathy involving the midfoot. J Foot Ankle Surg 2000;39:291–300.

[28] Rosenblum BI, Giurini JM, Miller LB, et al. Neuropathic ulcerations plantar to the lateral column in patients with Charcot foot deformity: a flexible approach to limb salvage. J Foot Ankle Surg 1997;36:360–3.
[29] Tom RK, Pupp GR. Talectomy for diabetic Charcot foot. An alternative to amputation. J Am Podiatr Med Assoc 1992;82:447–53.
[30] Barry DC, Sabacinski KA, Habershaw GM, et al. Tendoachilles procedures for chronic ulcerations in diabetic patients with transmetatarsal amputations. J Am Podiatr Med Assoc 1993;83: 96–100.

CLINICS IN PODIATRIC MEDICINE AND SURGERY

Clin Podiatr Med Surg 20 (2003) 793–801

Amputation considerations and energy expenditures in the diabetic patient

Kathleen Satterfield, DPM

Department of Orthopaedics, University of Texas Health Science Center at San Antonio, 7703 Floyd Curl Drive/ MS 7776, San Antonio, TX 78229, USA

Amputation has long been thought of as the white flag of diabetic foot care—the sign that the surgeon has lost hope and given up. It was generally assumed that one amputation would lead to successive, higher amputations and eventual disability and death. Only recently has it been realized that a minor, or even major, amputation may salvage the majority of the limb or save a life.

Though amputations still are undesired, they are at times unavoidable and even preferable to the need for chronic wound care, potential for infection, and the resulting need for higher level of amputation. At one time, surgeons treated amputations much like a gardener treated a tree with a broken, rotting limb. They simply looked at that segment in isolation, without regard to the rest of the tree, and severed the limb near the trunk. The gardener now has a tree with an exposed surface of wood that is discovered by parasites and insects that invade the tree. Because the tree is no longer symmetrical, when the spring winds blow, the weakened and infected tree is toppled.

The analogy can be made easily. The surgeon sees the necrotic hallux and resects it at the metatarsophalangeal joint. But the wound does not heal because there is insufficient circulation to meet the demands to heal it. Bacteria invade through the open wound and soon an infection is developing in the foot. The rigid foot type that led to the problem remains, and now, as the patient tries to walk without appropriate off-loading, tissues break down further. Infection, rigid deformity, and ischemia combine to topple the limb and perhaps even take the life of the patient.

Statistics of amputation

Few other disease states, unlike diabetes, are lightening rods for life-altering complications. Blindness, nephropathy, and amputation all conspire to limit the

E-mail address: satterfield@uthscsa.edu

doi:10.1016/S0891-8422(03)00074-0

independence of the patient who has diabetes. These complications are vastly out of proportion for the size of the population affected.

Less than 3% of the population in the United States has diabetes mellitus, yet more than 65% of all nontraumatic lower extremity amputations are secondary to the complications of the disease [1,2]. Statistics vary, but it is believed that between 5% and 15% of people who have diabetes will undergo a lower extremity amputation [3]. With the population growth continuing and the upsurge of minority immigrants, who have a higher incidence of diabetes, this complication will become endemic. It is imperative that foot surgeons do the appropriate planning for amputations to reduce the chance of successively higher levels of amputation.

Principles of amputation as limb salvage

Appropriate use of amputation as a tool to salvage the remainder of the limb requires close adherence to a set of principles that will improve the chances of long-term survival. These principles are as follows:

- Don't amputate as an isolated treatment.
- Do convert rigid deformities into flexible or low-pressure areas.
- Assess comorbidities that led to current condition and eliminate/control them.
- Remove all infected and marginal soft tissue and bone.
- Remove potentially dysvascular tissue.
- Plan the incision to accommodate for the possible need of further amputation.

Don't amputate as an isolated treatment

The nonviable ischemic digit does not present a dilemma to the surgeon who has no other option but to amputate. The challenge is to decide whether to amputate adjacent digits that may still be viable but challenge the functionality of the foot. A great number of amputation series begin with the hallux and first ray. Amputation at this level often solves an immediate problem of osteomyelitis. This is the pitfall of seeing a problem in isolation. The natural history of the hallux amputation was well documented in an article by Murdoch et al [4].

Findings of the retrospective study showed that in a series of 90 patients over a 10-year period, 60% had a subsequent second amputation, 21% had a third, and 7% had a fourth. The severity of the amputations that followed were notable, with 17% undergoing a below-the-knee amputation and 11% a transmetatarsal amputation on the same limb. There were also a number of contralateral amputations following the hallux amputation, including 3% below-knee level and 2% with transmetatarsal amputation. This progression is partially due to transference of deformity as patients develop rigid digital deformities at the interphalangeal and metarsophalangeal joints [3,5].

The amputation that is done as an isolated procedure is often one that will precipitate further procedures because of inattention to deforming tendinous and bony structures. Careful consideration of the various functions of the anatomic features of the lower extremity will lessen complications. In particular, the surgeon should not overlook the potential for a varus deformity that is possible after a Lisfranc's or a Chopart's amputation secondary to the anterior tibial tendon force and loss of the peroneal muscles' effects. This can either be redirected through a transposition of the anterior tibial tendon more laterally or transaction of the same tendon. If the latter course is taken, an ankle foot orthosis (AFO) will be required for active ambulation because of the loss of significant dorsiflexion at the ankle.

Attention should also be given to lengthening the Achilles tendon if there is distal forefoot pathology that could be minimized in the equines foot. This can easily be performed percutaneously.

Do convert rigid deformities

The rigid foot type is the most difficult to preserve if there is also neuropathy. Accommodative shoes and insoles provide only so much relief, and the comprehensive foot surgeon should assess the foot for surgical methods of converting a rigid deformity into a decreased area of force. Failure to do so either through conservative methods of shoeing or surgical means will not stand up to the rigors of ambulation with neuropathy.

If the distal forefoot is amputated, the mechanics for propelling the extremity forward transfer to the midfoot and rearfoot. Though this is truly an apropulsive gait, there is significant force generated to areas that have not previously had sustained focal force and this can lead to ulceration and eventually to amputation.

Assess comorbidities

Amputation in the diabetic foot is the result of infection, avascularity, or deformity. Because of the cascade of comorbidities experienced with diabetes, the surgeon must consider the medical aspects of the patient's condition with at least as much importance if not more than the technical aspects of the procedure.

Timing of the amputation in a patient with serious infection is never in question however. This is the first consideration with stabilization of comorbidities and vascular assessment to follow the life-saving amputation.

Anesthesia concerns are almost negated if spinal, regional, or local blocks are used instead of general anesthetic in the ill patient. A majority of the patients reaching this point also have severe neuropathy and may not require the level of anesthesia that the nondiabetic would.

Vascular disease, focal microvascular and macrovascular, must be assessed before the surgery in the case of the planned amputation. If the amputation is done on an emergent basis to prevent septicemia, the vascular testing can be postoperatively.

Infection and potential for septicemia far outweigh the potential for not healing at the level selected emergently for amputation. This is the surgical wound that will be revised, perhaps multiple times, and may be revascularized before final closure.

Elective procedures, such as tendon lengthenings are best left until the wound undergoes delayed primary closure because of potential complication of spread of infection.

It is important to realize that a palpable pedal pulse does not insure adequate circulation to heal an amputation site because it only shows circulation at that exact point. Calcification of vessels may not allow adequate perfusion to distal tissues. Inclusion of the full spectrum of noninvasive vascular testing will reveal macrovascular disease by Doppler pulse volume recordings, indicating significant level changes throughout the extremity; microvascular disease is revealed by transcutaneous oxygen perfusion.

Nutritional status is often overlooked but should be monitored by serum prealbumin and albumin levels, which should be 16 to 35 mg/dl and 3.5 to approximately 5 g/dl. Prealbumin indicates the immediate nutritional status, and the albumin represents that over a period of time. Though the patient who has diabetes may not be able to eat sufficient levels of protein without effecting diseased renal function, their nutritional status can be enhanced with supplements that aid in healing. Those most notably associated with wound healing include L-arginine and zinc.

Infection should be identified definitively through intraoperative cultures of deep tissue rather than surface cultures, which are often compromised by skin contaminants and colonized organisms.

Remove infected tissues

Failure to completely debride a site can doom a surgical wound to failure from the start. Necrotic tissue is clearly a risk if left, but the marginal tissues are the issue that the cautious surgeon sometimes hesitates to remove from the wound.

Debridement should be continued to the point at which unaffected tissue is visualized. Hemorrhagic vessels, fibrotic soft tissue, and discolored adipose all contribute to failure of a surgical procedure despite antibiotic therapy that might follow.

Remove potentially dysvascular tissue

Those tissues without a significant and independent blood supply should be removed from the wound at the time of the surgery. Potentially dysvascular tissue left in place becomes a nidus for infection as it degrades. Examples of potentially dysvascular tissue include tendons, capsules, plantar plates, and ligaments.

There is some controversy about removing cartilage of an opposing metatarsal after a digital amputation. The cartilage is dysvascular and may deteriorate without synovial fluid and a protective capsule. However, if the cartilage is removed during an initial procedure in an infected case, there is the potential of more proximal extension of infection through the denuded osseous structures.

Planning the incision

As multiple studies have shown, it is an unfortunate reality that one amputation may lead to another. The progressive nature of diabetes' complications, with increasing severity of vascular disease and neuropathy in particular, predisposes the patient to further procedures. The unfortunate occurrence is the need for more proximal amputation secondary to improper attention to the principles of amputation planning.

That planning extends to the realm of consideration that a subsequent surgery may be required at a later date. Incision planning must take into consideration the possible extension of amputation to the next level (ie, from an isolated ray to a transmetatarsal). Planning is most problematic when the presenting problem is an infected ulceration plantar to a metatarsal head that has now extended to a plantar space infection. This location of infection usually requires a Loeffler and Ballard incision [6]. This may be difficult to convert to a transmetatarsal amputation, if necessary, because of the curvilinear incision that extends from the metatarsal head and across the plantar surface to the medial foot to provide visual access to all of the compartments of the plantar foot. A key to being able to convert this to a proximal incision is to place the curvilinear incision adjacent to a metatarsal rather than directly beneath it and then carry it medially across the non–weight-bearing arch.

Rethinking amputations

Methods for amputation have been well described and there is little need for another detailed description of surgical techniques. But there is much need for decision criteria because surgeons continue to be resistant to the idea of amputation. Historically, the Syme amputation has not been a procedure performed by podiatric surgeons because of restrictive state laws that prevented amputation of the foot. This is changing, however, as multidisciplinary teams take to the operating room and as laws change. Therefore it is worthwhile to revisit the Syme amputation in more detail.

Syme amputation

In 1843 when James Syme first described the amputation that carries his name, he did not know that he was starting a controversy that would last into the twenty-first century. Few other procedures have been heralded, decried, and then rediscovered and praised so much as the Syme amputation.

The technique is to amputate at the level of the malleoli, which are removed at the level of the joint surface and closed. The two-stage procedure has historically been indicated for patients with significant disease in the forefoot, including suppuration, need for revascularization, severe rearfoot vascular status, and diabetes. There are now advocates for performing the Syme amputation in such patients [7].

This procedure involves removal of the forefoot by disarticulation at the level of the talus and dissection of the calcaneus from the surrounding soft tissues, retaining the neurovascular bundle that will supply it after closure. The malleoli are excised at a later date in the two-stage Syme. This surgical variation has been popularized by Michael Pinzur at Hines Veterans Administration Hospital [7]. Despite the revelations by Pinzur and others regarding the potential success of the Syme in patients who have diabetes, the patient with peripheral vascular disease and forefoot infection/tissue loss is more commonly advanced to a below-knee amputation. The vascular and orthopedic communities have lately advocated for a return to the Syme amputation, which could become a more mainstream alternative to below-knee amputation.

Guidelines for patient selection include need for an intact heel with sufficient soft tissue cover and a nonreconstructable forefoot [8]. At the University of Southern California Medical School Vascular Department, it is considered the amputation of choice in the dysvascular patient [9].

In one study, of the 29 patients who underwent successful Syme amputation, 28 were successfully rehabilitated. Thirteen were gait trained to walk unassisted, and 15 could ambulate with a cane or walker. This study included three patients who had a contralateral limb amputation. The one patient who had failure to rehabilitate died after a cardiac event [9].

Because this amputation is usually reserved for patients with comorbidities that contributed to their need for an amputation, they are predisposed to problems as the years advance. In Weaver's study of 29 successful Syme amputations in this population, four patients required revisional amputations secondary to two stump ulcerations, one with gangrene, and another with infection [9].

Given the high morbidity and mortality of this population, it has not always been clear why surgeons would opt for this procedure. The primary advantage that has been historically recognized is the patient's ability to transfer and walk without a prosthesis. The heel pad presents the surgeon with a thick skin surface with fat pad and mooring ligaments for stability [8,10].

Energy costs are important considerations in the population with cardiovascular insufficiencies. Because patients achieve a larger stride and faster pace with the Syme procedure, there is a lower energy expenditure when compared with the below-knee and especially the above-knee amputation [11].

Few patients with a Syme amputation remain unscathed as time continues, with many in the various reports developing contralateral amputations. The one complication that does not seem to develop in large numbers is ulceration secondary to neuropathy. In Weaver's study and in a large Hansen's disease study of neuropathic patients who had Syme amputation, the incidence of ulceration was remarkably low (below 15% in the Hansen's disease study and 0% in Weaver's study) [12].

Energy expenditures and rehabilitation potential

All levels of lower extremity amputation alter the function of the foot, demanding more of the proximal limb and increasing energy demands from the cardiovascular system. Many of the patients who have diabetes who require amputations already have significant vascular compromise throughout the body, and the new demands placed on the system by an amputation may prove to be too much.

A transmetatarsal amputation does not exclude the recipient from increased energy expenditures. It might be expected that less energy would be expended with this level of amputation because of the slower velocity of ambulation, a shorter limb reach, and a hind and midfoot [13–15]. The opposite is true, however. The decreased ability to generate adequate plantarflexory motion at the ankle creates the need to mobilize the extremity through hip muscles. The hip flexors essentially pull the extremity forward for ambulation [13].

The energy expenditure of the patient with a below-knee amputation is significantly higher though, and this is thought to be due to reduced propulsion from the prosthetic and gait asymmetry [16,17]. It is also a fact that the higher the amputation, the greater the energy expenditure [18]. It was historically accepted that the increase in energy was due to the weight of a prosthesis and the length of the residual limb, but this was disproved [19,20]. Instead, the socket shape appears to be the primary source of differences in metabolic expenditure [21].

Oxygen consumption rises significantly as a limb amputation is advanced proximally, from transtibial to transfemoral. At 2 km/h walking velocity, the volume of oxygen consumption in the transtibial amputee is 123% of that of the nonamputee. The transfemoral amputee rises to 155% of the nonamputee [18]. Oddly enough, assistive devices, such as crutches, canes, and walkers, actually raise the heart rate and energy use. This is because of the arm movements required to use the devices. Without these mobility tools, the patient will usually slow his pace to match his ability and this will reduce oxygen consumption, heart rate, and energy expenditure [18]. Therefore, there should be careful consideration before asking the patient to continue to ambulate with assistive devices after rehabilitation.

The role of race

It is well recognized that diabetes disproportionately affects African American, Hispanic, and Native American populations, but it is a recent discovery that ethnic minorities with diabetes mellitus have a significantly increased risk of amputation. This finding is independent of access to medical care, renal disease, hypertension, pulmonary disease, and cardiovascular disease [22].

In a retrospective study in the veterans health care system, the condition that was also prevalent in these minority groups who would go on to develop conditions leading to amputation was the presence of nephropathy [22]. Researchers recommend that minority patients with nephropathy be monitored carefully for development of foot problems.

In one study comparing amputation statistics in different ethnic groups, Young et al [22] reported that of veterans studied who had diabetes, Asians were more likely to have digital amputations, and Native American patients had a high percentage of below-knee amputations. Overall, Native Americans, although the smallest minority population, had the highest risk of amputation; African Americans had the second highest risk, followed by Hispanics, when compared with Caucasians.

Summary

Amputations are not procedures of choice but are often necessary and valuable tools for returning a patient to a more active lifestyle. Because of the comorbidities associated with diabetes, this is an important consideration. A return to a more active existence can reduce the effect of vascular disease, hyperglycemic states, and functional limitations.

It is an interesting and not uncommon occurrence for the chronic wound patient, when offered an amputation, to have the procedure because the frequency of needed medical care has stripped him of his independence. The frequency of wound care in the nonhealing wound and its personal demands can be compared with the demands placed on the dialysis patient.

The greatest obstacle for the uninitiated surgeon is a sense of hesitancy: Am I moving too fast to amputation as an answer? The ability to make this decision comes with experience and with prioritizing the patient's needs. Life-threatening infections and avascular extremities that are not bypassable are the easier decisions to make, as there is little choice at that point.

In deciding whether to amputate, the wise surgeon will take into consideration the medical and mobility needs of each patient and determine level and timing based on understanding of the whole person.

References

[1] Reiber GE, Boyko EJ, Smith DG. Lower extremity foot ulcers and amputations in diabetes. Diabetes in America. Washington, DC: National Institutes of Health; National Institute of Diabetes and Digestive and Kidney Diseases; 1995. p. 349–85. Publication #NIH 95–1468.
[2] Reiber GE. Epidemiology and health care cost for diabetic foot problems. In: LoGerfo FW, editor. Diabetic foot: medical and surgical management. Totowa (NJ): Human Press; 2002. p. 35–8.
[3] Lavery L, Lavery D, Quebedeaux T. Increased foot pressures after great toe amputation in diabetes. Diabetes Care 1995;18:1460–2.
[4] Murdoch DP, et al. The natural history of great toe amputations. J Foot Ankle Surg 1997;36: 204–9.
[5] Quebedeaux T, Lavery L, Lavery D. The development of foot deformity and ulcers after great toe amputation in diabetes. Diabetes Care 1996;19:165–7.
[6] Loeffler RD, Ballard A. Plantar fascial spaces of the foot and a proposed surgical approach. Foot Ankle 1980;1(1):11–4.
[7] Pinzur MS, Morrison C, Sage R, et al. Syme's two-stage amputation in insulin-requiring diabetics with gangrene of the forefoot. Foot Ankle 1991;11:394–6.

[8] Wagner FW. The Syme amputation. In: Atlas of limb prosthetics: surgical and prosthetic principles. St. Louis (MO): CV Mosby; 1981. p. 326–40.
[9] Weaver FA, Modrall JG, Baek S, et al. Syme amputation: results in patients with severe forefoot ischemia. Cardiovasc Surg 1996;4:81–6.
[10] Francis H, Roberts JR, Clagett GP, et al. Syme amputation: success in elderly diabetic patients with palpable ankle pulse. J Vasc Surg 1990;12:237–40.
[11] Rutherford RB, Flanigan DPO, Gupta SG, et al. Suggested standard for reports dealing with lower extremity ischemia. J Vasc Surg 1986;4:80–94.
[12] Srinivasan H. Syme's amputation in insensitive feet. J Bone Joint Surg 1973;55:558–62.
[13] Garbalosa JC, Cavanagh PR, Wu G, et al. Foot function in diabetic patients after partial amputation. Foot Ankle Int 1996;17:43–8.
[14] Mueller MJ, Salsich GB, Bastian AJ. Differences in the gait characteristics of people with diabetes and transmetatarsal amputation compared with age-matched controls. Gait Posture 1998;7:200–6.
[15] Mueller MJ, Salsich GB, Strube MJ. Functional limitations in patients with diabetes and transmetatarsal amputation. Phys Ther 1997;77:937–43.
[16] Huang CT, Jackson JR, Moore NB, et al. Amputation: energy cost of ambulation. Arch Phys Med Rehabil 1979;60:19–24.
[17] Waters RL, Perry J, Antoneli D, Hislop H. Energy cost of walking of amputees: the influence of level amputation. J Bone Surg Am 1976;58:42–8.
[18] Waters RL, Mulroy S. The energy expenditure of normal and pathological gait. Gait Posture 1999;9(3):207–31.
[19] Gailey RS, Nash M, Atchley T, et al. The effects of prosthesis mass on metabolic cost of ambulation in non-vascular trans-tibial amputees. Prosthet Orthot Int 1997;21(1):9–16.
[20] Gailey RS, Wenger M, Raya M, et al. Energy expenditure of trans-tibial amputees during ambulation at self-selected pace. Prosthet Orthot Int 1994;18(2):84–91.
[21] Gailey RS, Lawrence D, Bburditt C, et al. The CAT-CAM socket and quadrilateral socket: a comparison of energy cost during ambulation. Prosthet Orthot Int 1993;17(2):95–100.
[22] Young BA, Maynard C, Boyko EJ. Racial differences in diabetic neuropathy, cardiovascular disease and mortality in a national population of veterans. Diabetes Care 2003;26:2392–9.

Clin Podiatr Med Surg
20 (2003) 803–824

CLINICS IN PODIATRIC MEDICINE AND SURGERY

Cumulative Index 2003

Volume 20

January	EXTERNAL FIXATION OF THE FOOT AND ANKLE, pages 1–198
April	PERIOPERATIVE MANAGEMENT OF THE PODIATRIC PATIENT, pages 199–372
July	CLINICAL PODOGERIATRICS: ASSESSMENT, EDUCATION AND PREVENTION, pages 373–634
October	DIABETES MELLITUS, pages 635–824

Note: Page numbers of article titles are in **boldface** type.

A

Abductor digiti minimi flap, in diabetic foot reconstruction, 779

Abductor hallucis flap, in diabetic foot reconstruction, 778

Ablative surgery, in diabetic foot, 720–721

ABLE (Althof-Beasley Lower Extremity Presurgical Assessment Tool), for psychological management, 204–208

Abscess, subungual, 432

Acarbose, for diabetes mellitus, 221–222, 643

Accidents, risk assessment for, in long-term care, 392

Acetaminophen, for diabetic neuropathy, 679

Acetohexamide, for diabetes mellitus, 640–641

Achilles tendon
- anatomy of, 362
- insertion tendinosis of, retrocalcaneal exostectomy for, **361–366**
- lengthening of, in diabetes mellitus, 790

Advanced glycation end products, in diabetes mellitus, 677

Age considerations, in external fixation, 22

Akin osteotomy, external fixation for, 35–36

Allopurinol, for gout, 483

Alpha-glucosidase inhibitors, for diabetes mellitus, 221–222, 643

Alpha-methyl dopa, preoperative evaluation of, 225

Alternative medications, preoperative evaluation of, 232–234

Althof-Beasley Lower Extremity Presurgical Assessment Tool, for psychological management, 204–208

Amantadine, for diabetic neuropathy, 683

American Society of Anesthesiologists, surgical risk categories of, 616–617

Amikacin, for diabetic foot infections, 664

Amitriptyline, for diabetic neuropathy, 680–681

Amoxicillin/clavulanate, for diabetic foot infections, 659–660

Ampicillin, for diabetic foot infections, 664

Ampicillin/sulbactam, for diabetic foot infections, 659–660, 662–664

Amputation
- in Charcot foot, 747
- in diabetic foot, 399, 611–612, 720–721, **793–801**
  - comorbidity assessment in, 795–796
  - debridement with, 796
  - dysvascular tissue removal in, 796–797
  - energy expenditures after, 799
  - epidemiology of, 710
  - in comprehensive treatment plan, 794–795

doi:10.1016/S0891-8422(03)00101-0

in infections, 665
in limb salvage, 794–797
incision planning in, 797
indications for, 793
prevention of. *See* Surgery, for diabetic foot, elective.
racial factors in, 799–800
rethinking, 797
rigid deformities and, 795
risk factors for, 783–784
statistics of, 793–794
Syme, 797–798
in severe trauma, versus salvage, 301

Analgesia, perioperative
epidural, cryotherapy effects on, 263–264
patient-controlled, 262
preemptive, **237–255**
spinal, 263–264

Anesthesia
for extracorporeal shock wave therapy, for plantar fasciitis, 329
for trauma repair, 300–301

Angiography, in arterial occlusive disease, in diabetes mellitus, 699–702

Angioplasty, of peripheral vessels, in diabetes mellitus, 702–704

Angiotensin-converting enzyme inhibitors
for diabetic neuropathy, 683
preoperative evaluation of, 226

Ankle
arthrodesis of, in degenerative disease, 345–346
Charcot. *See* Charcot foot and ankle.
external fixation applications in, **65–96**
arthrodesis, 164–169
tibiocalcaneal, 16, 85–89
tibiotalar, 16, 74–85
triple, 16, 89–90
biomechanics of, 67–69
capabilities of, 66
circular, 67–69
complications of, 92–93
distraction arthrodiastasis, 90–92
frame removal in, 94
limitations of, 66–67
wire considerations in, 69–74

Ankle block, in trauma, 298

Ankle joint replacement, case review of, **335–359**
discussion, 342–349, 357
history of injury, 336–337, 350–352
physical examination, 337–339
postoperative course, 340–342, 355–356
procedure, 339–340

Anonychia, 431

Antiarrhythmic agents, for diabetic neuropathy, 682

Antibiotics, for diabetic foot infections, 658–665, 719

Anticoagulants
for deep venous thrombosis prophylaxis, 277–279
preoperative evaluation of, 226–229

Anticonvulsants, for diabetic neuropathy, 681–682

Antidepressants
for diabetic neuropathy, 680–681
preoperative evaluation of, 231

Antiplatelet agents, preoperative evaluation of, 230

Antipsychotics, preoperative evaluation of, 231

Anxiety, foot pain in, 401

Anxiolytics, preoperative evaluation of, 231

AO/ASIF system, for subtalar arthrodesis. *See* Synthes tubular external fixation.

Argatroban, for deep venous thrombosis, 278–279

Arterial occlusive disease
in diabetes mellitus, **689–708**
amputation risk in, 784
arterial reconstruction in, 702–704
evaluation of
angiography in, 699–701
Doppler studies in, 697–699
exercise testing in, 696
general assessment in, 690–691
limb pressure measurements in, 693–695
magnetic resonance imaging in, 701–702
physical examination in, 691–693
pulse volume recordings in, 695–696
toe pressure measurements in, 695
transcutaneous oximetry in, 696–697
pathophysiology of, 689
treatment of, 702–704, 719
in elderly persons
healing ability and, 531–532
history of, 527–532
noninvasive evaluation of, 539–543

physical examination in, 532–538
risk factors for, 530–531

Arterial ulcers, in elderly persons, 389, 399

Arthritis
degenerative. *See* Osteoarthritis.
in elderly persons, **469–485**
biomechanics of, 470–472
diagnosis of, 378
epidemiology of, 469–470
flatfoot in, 502
gout, 481–483
hallux rigidus in, 491–493
osteoarthritis. *See* *under* Osteoarthritis.
psoriatic, 462–463
reactive versus nonreactive joints in, 472–473
rheumatoid, 477–481
treatment of, 472–474
types of, 469
rheumatoid. *See* Rheumatoid arthritis.

Arthrodesis
ankle, in degenerative disease, 345–346
external fixation for
ankle, 164–169
calcaneocuboid, 54–56
first metatarsocuneiform, 33–35
first metatarsophalangeal, 30–32
naviculocuneiform, 57–58
subtalar, **181–194**
talonavicular, 56–57
tarsometatarsal, 52–54
tibiocalcaneal, 16, 85–89
tibiotalar, 16, 74–85
triple, 16, 89–90
for Charcot foot, 751–752

Arthrodiastasis, distraction, 90–92

Arthrometric examination, of deformities, 514–515

Arthropathy, Charcot. *See* Charcot foot and ankle.

Arthroplasty, hallux, in diabetes mellitus, 786–787

Arthrosis, post-traumatic, ankle joint replacement for, case review of, **335–359**

Aspirin
for deep venous thrombosis, 282
preoperative evaluation of, 230–232

Assessment, of elderly persons, 378–379, **407–429**
clinical findings, 413–414
for accident risk, in long-term care, 392
for biomechanical conditions, 417–418
for chronic diseases, 411–412
for diabetes mellitus, **573–582**
for pressure ulcers, 384–385
in long-term care, 383–389
initial, 408–414
Medicare class findings in, 414–415
Medicare codes and, 408–411
neurological, **547–571**
outline for, 416–417
preoperative, 619–621
protocol for, 418–424
symptoms, 412–413
systems review in, 408

Association for the Study of Internal Fixation (AO/ASIF), fracture management principles of, 292–293

Atenolol, preoperative evaluation of, 225

Atherosclerosis, in peripheral vascular disease, 530, 690–691

Autonomic dysfunction, assessment of, in diabetes mellitus, 713

Avulsion, of nail, 434

Aztreonam, for diabetic foot infections, 664

B

Babinski's sign, in neurological evaluation, 567

Balance realignment therapy, for deformities, 521

Beau's lines, 436

Becaplermin, for diabetic ulcers, 717

Benzodiazepines
for diabetic neuropathy, 679
preoperative evaluation of, 231

Beta-blockers, preoperative evaluation of, 224–225

Beta-lactamase inhibitors, for diabetic foot infections, 663

Betacarotene, for warts, 464

Biguanides, for diabetes mellitus, 222, 641–642

Bilobed flaps, in diabetic foot reconstruction, 767–769

Biomechanics
of arthritis, 470–472
of deformities, evaluation of, 512–518
of diabetic foot, 575–576
of hyperkeratosis formation, 444–445

Biopsy
of bone, in osteomyelitis, in diabetes mellitus, 658–659
of skin lesions, 454–456

Bisoprolol, preoperative evaluation of, 225

Blisters, 385, 464–465

Block balance testing, for deformities, 521–523

Blood vessels, injury of, in external fixation, 92

Bone
biopsy of, in osteomyelitis, in diabetes mellitus, 658–659
destructive changes of, in diabetes mellitus. *See* Charcot foot and ankle.

Bone block distraction, in calcaneocuboid joint arthrodesis, 54–56

Bone graft, external fixation for, 36

Bone scan, in diabetic foot, 732–735
with osteoarthropathy, 657
with ulcers, 714–715

Brachymetatarsal, correction of, external fixation for, 36–38

Braden Scale, for pressure ulcer staging, 385

Brief Pain Inventory, 258

Buechel-Pappas ankle prosthesis, 339–340, 348–349, 351–356

Bullous diseases, 464–465

Bunion. *See* Hallux valgus.

Bunionette (tailor's bunion), 497–498

Bupivacaine, for preemptive analgesia, 246

Bursitis, retrocalcaneal, retrocalcaneal exostectomy for, **361–366**

C

Calcaneocuboid joint, arthrodesis of, external fixation for, 54–56

Calcaneus
fractures of, external fixation for, 169–170
spurs on, retrocalcaneal exostectomy for, **361–366**

Callus (tyloma), 397–398, 445

Callus distraction, external fixation for, 19

Cancer, skin, in elderly persons, 463–464

Capsaicin
for diabetic neuropathy, 682–683
for osteoarthritis, 476

Carbamazepine, for diabetic neuropathy, 681

Cardiovascular drugs, preoperative evaluation of, 224–226

Cardiovascular system, preoperative evaluation of, 214

Cast
for Charcot foot, 747
total-contact, for diabetic ulcers, 718
versus external fixation, 13

Cavovarus foot, external fixation for, 49

Cavus foot, 503–505
midfoot osteotomy for, external fixation for, 58–59

Cefadroxil, for diabetic foot infections, 659–660

Cefazolin, for diabetic foot infections, 658

Cefepime, for diabetic foot infections, 659, 662, 664

Cefoperazone, for diabetic foot infections, 664

Cefotaxime, for diabetic foot infections, 664

Cefoxitin, for diabetic foot infections, 662–663

Ceftazidime, for diabetic foot infections, 662–664

Ceftriaxone, for diabetic foot infections, 662–663

Celecoxib, for perioperative pain, preemptive administration of, 250

Cephalexin, for diabetic foot infections, 659

Cerebellar function, assessment of, 568–569

Charcot foot and ankle, **97–117, 741–756**
acute
diagnosis of, 746
treatment of, 747–751
chronic, treatment of, 751–754
classification of, 730, 744–746
clinical features of, 730
definition of, 97
diagnosis of, 746
differential diagnosis of, 730
etiology of, 741–742
external fixation for, 19, 49–52, 59–60, 747–753
goals of, 98–100
postoperative care in, 112–116
surgical options in, 101–103
techniques for, 104–112

imaging in, 656–658, **729–740**
in diabetes mellitus, 578
incidence of, 97–98
pathophysiology of, 729–730, 742–743
stages of, 98
treatment of, 743–744, 747, 789–790

Charnley, J.C., external fixation devices of, 5

Charnley classification, of foot and ankle trauma, 298

Chlorpropamide, for diabetes mellitus, 640–641

Ciprofloxacin, for diabetic foot infections, 659–660, 662, 664–665

Claudication, intermittent, in peripheral vascular disease, 527–529, 690

Claw toes, 489–491

Clinafloxacin, for diabetic foot infections, 660

Clindamycin, for diabetic foot infections, 659–660, 662, 664–665

Clonidine
for diabetic neuropathy, 683
preoperative evaluation of, 225

Clopidogrel, preoperative evaluation of, 230

Closed reduction, in Charcot foot, 749, 751

Clots, deep venous. *See* Deep venous thrombosis.

Clubbing, of nails, 432

Clubfoot, correction of, external fixation for, 17–18

Coagulation disorders
deep venous thrombosis in, 271
from alternative medications, 232–233

Colchicine, for gout, 482

Cold therapy. *See* Cryotherapy.

Collagen dressing, for diabetic ulcers, 717

Coma, in diabetes mellitus, 639

Compartment syndrome, in ankle trauma, 295–296

Complementary medications, preoperative evaluation of, 232–234

Comprehensive care plans, for nursing home residents, 389

Compression, in forefoot applications, external fixation for, 30–36

Computed tomography
in deep venous thrombosis, 275, 280
in diabetic foot, 737
in diabetic foots, with osteoarthropathy, 657–658

Computer-assisted sensory examination, in diabetes mellitus, 675

Computerized blood flow studies, in diabetic foot, 734

Confusion, postoperative, 623

Congenital nail disorders, 432

Contact dermatitis, 459–460

Contractures, in trauma, external fixation for, 174, 176

Contusions, of nail plate, 434

Corn
hard (heloma durum), 445
nail bed, 434, 445
seed (heloma miliare), 445
soft (heloma molle), 446

Coronary artery disease, peripheral vascular disease and, 530

Corticosteroids
for skin disorders, 461–462
intraarticular
for gout, 482
for osteoarthritis, 477
for rheumatoid arthritis, 480
preoperative evaluation of, 230

Cranial neuropathy, in diabetes mellitus, 674

Cryotherapy, postoperative, **307–322**
continuous-flow
case reports on, 311–314
normal subject trials of, 314–319
prescription for, 319–320
injury from, 310–311
pain physiology and, 307–310

Culture, in infections, in diabetes mellitus, 656, 719

Curative surgery, in diabetic foot, 720

Custom-molded footwear, for elderly persons, 593, 595, 598, 600

Cyclooxygenase inhibitors, for perioperative pain, 250, 260

D

D-dimer degradation products, in deep venous thrombosis, 275–276

Dalteparin, for deep venous thrombosis, 278

Debridement
in trauma, 299–300, 302

of diabetic foot infections, 665, 716
of pressure ulcers, 386

Deep venous thrombosis, in surgery, **269–289**
anatomic considerations in, 272
case reviews of, 283–285
diagnosis of, 274–276
epidemiology of, 269
for trauma, 300, 304–305
natural history of, 271–272
pathophysiology of, 270–272
prophylaxis for, 228–229, 276–277, 281–283, 300
risk factors for, 269–270, 272–273, 281
treatment of, 277–280

Deformities
external fixation correction of, 16–18
in midfoot, 47–49
lower leg. *See* Lower leg deformities.
in diabetes mellitus
elective reconstruction of, 720–721
surgical treatment of. *See* Surgery, for diabetic foot, elective.
treatment of, 795
ulcers in, 711–713, 720–721
in elderly persons, **487–509, 511–526**
biomechanical evaluation of, 512–518
claw toes, 489–491
compensatory malalignments in, 518–519
footwear for, 523–526, 595–596. *See also* Footwear.
hallux rigidus, 491–493
hallux valgus. *See* Hallux valgus.
hammertoes, 487–491
heel pain, 505–508
in diabetes mellitus, 575
in osteoarthritis, 475–476
metatarsalgia, 498–501
orthoses for, 523–526. *See also* Orthoses.
pain in, 398
pathomechanics of, 518–523
pes cavus, 503–505
pes planus, 501–503
surgery for, 610–611
tailor's bunion, 497–498

Delirium, postoperative, 623

Depression, surgical outcome and, 202

Dermatitis, contact, 459–460

Dermatitis herpetiformis, 465

Dermis, tissue-engineered, for diabetic ulcers, 717–718

Desipramine, for diabetic neuropathy, 680

Diabetes mellitus, **635–653**
amputation in. *See* Amputation, in diabetic foot.
Charcot foot and ankle in. *See* Charcot foot and ankle.
classification of, 636
diagnosis of, 637
epidemiology of, 671
imaging in, 656–658, **729–740**
in elderly persons
assessment of, **573–582**
diagnosis of, 379–380
nail disorders in, 437
onychopathy in, 397
osteoarthritis in, 474–475
pain in, 398–399
patient education on, 574
peripheral neuropathy in, 574–575, 578
preventive care in, **573–582**
surgical management in, 611–612
surgical risks in, 615–616
ulcers in
assessment of, 573–582
in long-term care, 383–384, 387–388, 393–394
pain in, 399
prevention of, 573–582
incidence of, 635
infections in, **655–669**
morbidity and mortality in, 671, 709–710
pathogenesis of, 637–638
peripheral neuropathy in, **671–688**
preoperative considerations with, 215, 219–224
screening for, 637
signs and symptoms of, 638–639
soft tissue reconstruction in, **757–781**
surgery in, **783–792**
treatment of
alpha glucosidase inhibitors in, 643
biguanides in, 641–642
combination, 644
glucose monitoring in, 647
hypoglycemia in, 649
in neuropathy, 677–678
insulin for, 644–647
meglitinides in, 643–644
oral hypoglycemic drugs in, 639–640
perioperative, 647–649
sulfonylureas in, 640–641
thiazolidinediones in, 642
ulcers in, **709–728**
vascular disorders in, **689–708**
versus normal insulin metabolism and glucose homeostasis, 637

Diabetic lumbosacral radiculoplexus neuropathy, 673–674

Dicloxacillin, for diabetic foot infections, 659

Digit(s). *See* Toe(s).

Digital artery island flaps, in diabetic foot reconstruction, 772, 774

Diphenhydramine, for diabetic neuropathy, 679

Disease-modifying antirheumatic drugs, for rheumatoid arthritis, 479–480

Distraction
- arthrodiastasis, 90–92
- in forefoot applications, external fixation for, 36–40

Diuretics, preoperative evaluation of, 226

Doppler studies, in peripheral vascular disease
- in diabetes mellitus, 697–699, 713
- in elderly persons, 539–540

Dornier Epos Ultra device, for plantar fasciitis, 326, 329–330

Dorsalis pedis pulse, evaluation of, in peripheral vascular disease, 533–534

Double-Z rhomboid flaps, in diabetic foot reconstruction, 769–770, 772–773

Dressings
- for diabetic ulcers, 717–718
- for pressure ulcers, 385–387

Drug(s)
- interactions of, in elderly persons, 376
- preoperative evaluation of. *See* Preoperative evaluation, of medications.

Dynafix external fixation system, for forefoot, 27–29

Dynamization, in external fixation, 21

E

Eccrine poroma, 446

Edema, in external fixation, 22

Elderly persons
- arthritis in. *See* Arthritis, in elderly persons.
- atypical illness presentation in, 375–376
- care of, principles of, **373–381**
- deformities in, **487–509, 511–526**
- demographics of, 373
- diabetes mellitus in. *See* Diabetes mellitus, in elderly persons.
- external fixation in, 22
- footwear for, 387, 576, **593–605**
- heterogeneity of, 374
- hyperkeratotic lesions in. *See* Hyperkeratosis, in elderly persons.
- interrelated health events in, 374
- long-term care of, **383–394,** 585
- multidisciplinary care of, 377–378
- multiple conditions in, 375
- nail disorders in. *See* Nail disorders, in elderly persons.
- neurologic evaluation in, **547–571,** 616
- pain in. *See* Pain, in elderly persons.
- peripheral neuropathy in, 379, 574–575, 578
- peripheral vascular disease in. *See* Peripheral vascular disease, in elderly persons.
- podiatric assessment in, 378–379, 383–389, **407–429**
- polypharmacy in, 376
- preoperative evaluation of, 217
- primary care of, **583–591**
- skin disorders in. *See* Skin disorders, in elderly persons.
- surgical considerations in. *See* Surgery, in elderly persons.
- treatment goals for, 377

Electrohydraulic principle, in shock wave generation, 326

Electromagnetic principle, in shock wave generation, 326

Electrophysiologic studies, in diabetes mellitus, 675–676

Elevation dependency test, in peripheral vascular disease, 534–535

Embolism, pulmonary, in deep venous thrombosis, 270–272, 274

Emotional disorders, manifested in foot, 400

Endocrine disorders, preoperative evaluation of, 215

Endothelial injury, deep venous thrombosis in, 270–271

Endovascular therapy, for vascular disease, in diabetes mellitus, 704

Energy expenditures, after amputation, in diabetes mellitus, 799

Enoxaparin, for deep venous thrombosis, 278

Ephedra, preoperative evaluation of, 234

Epidural analgesia, cryotherapy effects on, 263–264

Epinephrine, in local anesthetics, duration of action with, 245

Epos Ultra device, for plantar fasciitis, 326, 329–330

Equinus deformity
external fixation for, 49
in Charcot foot, 99

Ertapenem, for diabetic foot infections, 662

Exercise, for osteoarthritis, 476

Exercise testing, in peripheral vascular disease, 696

Exostectomy, retrocalcaneal, **361–366**

Exostosis
retrocalcaneal, retrocalcaneal exostectomy for, **361–366**
subungual, 434

Extensor digitorum brevis flap, in diabetic foot reconstruction, 777

External fixation
advantages of, 12–13, 66
complications of, 20–22
in forefoot applications, 40
in rearfoot applications, 92–93
disadvantages of, 13–14
in forefoot applications, 30
in rearfoot applications, 66–67
for Charcot foot reconstruction. *See* Charcot foot and ankle, external fixation for.
for deformity correction, 16–18, 47–49, **119–157**
for subtalar arthrodesis, **181–194**
for trauma, 15–16, 35, 47–49, **159–180**
forefoot applications of, **27–44**
fracture after, 21
history of, **1–8,** 9–11, 119, 125, 127
indications for, 14–20, 46–47, 180
midfoot applications of, **45–63**
monolateral devices for, 11
patient selection for, 22–24
psychologic issues in, 23–24
rearfoot applications of, **97–117**
removal of, 21
ring devices for, 11
self-care in, 22–23
training for, 11–12, 14
types of, 11–12, 127, 129

Extracorporeal shock wave therapy, **323–334**
approved devices for, 326
for nonunion, 332
for plantar fasciitis, 326–332
historical review of, 323–324
physics of, 324
physiologic effects of, 324–325
wave generation in, 325–326

F

Factor V Leiden gene mutation, deep venous thrombosis in, 271

Falls, risk assessment for, in long-term care, 392

Fasciotomy, plantar fasciitis, 328

Femoral pulse, evaluation of, in peripheral vascular disease, 533–534

Femoropopliteal reconstruction and bypass, in diabetes mellitus, 702–703

Fibula, fractures of, joint replacement for, case review of, **335–359**

First ray, ulceration at, in diabetes mellitus, surgery for, 786–787

Flaps, in diabetic foot reconstruction, 21, 761–779
local random, 761–773
advancement, 763
advantages of, 761
anatomic considerations in, 762–763
bilobed, 767–769
definition of, 761
double-Z rhomboid, 769–770, 772–773
rhomboid, 769
rotation, 764–765
transposition, 764–766
types of, 761–762
muscle, 21–23, 775
pedicle, 771, 773–779
digital artery island, 774
instep (medial plantar artery), 774
reverse flow sural artery neuro-fasciocutaneous, 774–776

Flatfoot, 501–503

Flexor digitorum brevis flap, in diabetic foot reconstruction, 778

Fluoxetine, for diabetic neuropathy, 680–681

Food and Drug Administration, shock wave devices approved by, 326

Footwear
for Charcot foot, 747, 751
for diabetic foot, 722
inspection of, 713
ulcerated, 718
for elderly persons, **593–605**
appropriate for activity, 594
construction of, 594–595
custom-molded, 593, 595, 598, 600
hallux valgus due to, 493–494
in claw toe deformity, 490
in deformities, 523–526
in diabetic ulcers, 387, 576
in hallux rigidus, 492–493
in hallux valgus, 495–497
in hammertoe deformity, 490
in metatarsalgia, 499–500

in pes cavus, 505
in pes planus, 503
in plantar heel pain, 506–507
Medicare coverage of, 593
modifications for, 595–598
selection of, 599–600

Forefoot, external fixation applications in, **27–44**
bone grafts, 36
brachymetatarsal correction, 36–38
complications in, 40
compression, 30–36
devices for, 27–30
distraction, 36–40
first metatarsocuneiform joint arthrodesis, 33–35
first metatarsophalangeal joint arthrodesis, 30–32
fractures, 35
Freiberg's disease, 39–40
hallux limitus/rigidus, 39
management in, 40–41
osteotomy, 35–36
shortened first metatarsal, 38–39
soft tissue contraction, 40

Foreign bodies, in nail plate, 435

Fracture(s)
ankle joint replacement for, case review of, **335–359**
external fixation for
calcaneal, 169–170
Lisfranc's, 47–49
metatarsal, 35, 169–172, 174–175
open, 15–16
phalanges, 170–172, 174–175
pilon, 15
talar, 160, 162–166, 169
tibial, 160, 162–166
nonunion of, extracorporeal shock wave therapy for, 332

Freiberg's disease, external fixation for, 39–40

Fungal infections, in elderly persons, 466

G

Gabapentin, for diabetic neuropathy, 681–682

Gait, assessment of
in biomechanical evaluation, 517–518
in neurological evaluation, 551–552

Garlic, preoperative evaluation of, 233

Geriatric patients. *See* Elderly persons.

Ginkgo, preoperative evaluation of, 233

Ginseng, preoperative evaluation of, 233

Glimepiride, for diabetes mellitus, 220, 641

Glipizide, for diabetes mellitus, 220, 641, 644

Glitazones, for diabetes mellitus, 642

Glucosamine, for osteoarthritis, 476

Glucose
homeostasis of, 637
monitoring of, in diabetes mellitus, 647

Glucosidase inhibitors, for diabetes mellitus, 221–222, 643

Glyburide, for diabetes mellitus, 220, 641, 644

Gosnell Scale, for pressure ulcer staging, 385

Gout, in elderly persons, 398, 481–483

Graphesthesia, assessment of, 558

Growth factors, for diabetic ulcers, 717

Guanabenz, preoperative evaluation of, 225

Guanfacine, preoperative evaluation of, 225

Gustillo and Anderson classification, of foot and ankle trauma, 298

H

Haglund's deformity, retrocalcaneal exostectomy for, **361–366**

Half-pin fixator, for tibiotalar arthrodesis, 82, 84–85

Hallux, arthroplasty of, in diabetes mellitus, 786–787

Hallux limitus, 39, 398

Hallux rigidus, 398, 491–493
external fixation for, 39

Hallux valgus, 493–497
biomechanics of, 472
causes of, 493–495
pain in, 398
surgery for, 609
treatment of, 495–497

Hammertoes, 487–491, 785–786

Hapalonychia, 436

Hard corn (heloma durum), 445

Hawkins classification, of foot and ankle trauma, 298

Healing
in elderly persons
factors affecting, 457–458
nutrition for, 458–459, 532, 620–621
of surgical wounds, 616, 622–623
of diabetic ulcers, 715–719, 758

HealthTronics Ossatron device, for plantar fasciitis, 326

Heel
in footwear, modifications of, 597
reconstruction of, in diabetes mellitus, 789–790

Heel pain
plantar, 505–508. *See also* Plantar fasciitis.
retrocalcaneal exostectomy for, **361–366**

Heloma
pain in, 397–398
subungual, 434, 445

Heloma durum (hard corn), 445

Heloma miliare (seed corn), 445

Heloma molle (soft corn), 446

Heloma neurofibrosum, 446

Heloma vasculare, 446

Heparin
for deep venous thrombosis, 277–278
preoperative evaluation of, 228–229

Herbal medications, preoperative evaluation of, 232–234

Hindfoot. *See* Rearfoot.

Hirudin, for deep venous thrombosis, 279

Hives, 460

Hoffman, Raoul, external fixation devices of, 4, 11

Home care, foot care in, 393–394

Hyaluronic acid products, for osteoarthritis, 477

Hydrocodone, for diabetic neuropathy, 680

Hydromorphone, for trauma, 299

Hyperbaric oxygen therapy, for diabetic ulcers, 719

Hypercoagulable states, deep venous thrombosis in, 271, 280

Hyperglycemia, in diabetes mellitus, 639
polyneuropathy development in, 674, 676–677

Hyperkeratosis, in elderly persons, **443–452**
biomechanics of, 444–445
causes of, 444–445
classification of, 443–444
diagnosis of, 447
pain in, 397–398
patient education on, 448
subungual, 434, 437
symptoms of, 445–447
treatment of, 447–448, 584

Hypermobility, of joints, 473–474

Hyperpigmentation, of nail plate, 437

Hypertension, surgical risks in, 615

Hyperuricemia, gout in, 481–483

Hypoglycemia, in diabetes mellitus, treatment of, 649

I

Ibuprofen, for diabetic neuropathy, 679

Ilizarov, Gavriel A., external fixation devices of, 6–8, 77–82, 119, 125, 127

Imaging. *See specific modalities.*

Imipenem, for diabetic foot infections, 664

Imipramine, for diabetic neuropathy, 680–681

Immobilization, in Charcot foot, 747

Immunosuppressive therapy, for rheumatoid arthritis, 480

Infections
in ankle trauma, 294
in diabetes mellitus, **655–669**
antibiotics for, 658–665
costs of, 666
culture in, 656, 719
evaluation of, 655–656
imaging in, 656–658, 729–740
in elderly persons, 577–578
in ulcers, 714
laboratory testing in, 656
pathogens causing, 658
recommendations for, 665–666
surgery for, 665
treatment of, 718–719, 795–796
in elderly persons, 466
in diabetes mellitus, 577–578
of nails, 432
of pressure ulcers, 387
in external fixation, 13, 21, 93, 176–177
local anesthetic failure in, 245

Inflammation
cryotherapy effects on, 309
of nails, 432

Informed consent, for surgery, in elderly persons, 621

Ingrown nails, in diabetes mellitus, 785–786

Injury. *See* Trauma.

Instep (medial plantar artery) flaps, in diabetic foot reconstruction, 774

Insulin
for diabetes mellitus
perioperative, 648–649
regimens for, 646–647
types of, 644–646
metabolism of, 637
preoperative evaluation of, 222–224

Insulin secretagogues, preoperative evaluation of, 221

Intermittent claudication, in peripheral vascular disease, 527–529

Internal fixation
of ankle fractures, arthrosis after, joint replacement for, **335–359**
versus external fixation, 13–14

Interphalangeal joint(s)
first, arthroplasty of, in diabetes mellitus, 786
hammertoe deformity involving, 487–491

Intramedullary nails, for Charcot foot, 751

Irrigation, wound, in trauma, 299–300

Ischemic vascular disease. *See* Peripheral vascular disease.

Island flaps, in diabetic foot reconstruction, 772, 774

J

Joint(s)
Charcot. *See* Charcot foot and ankle.
subluxation of, in external fixation, 22

K

Kaposi's sarcoma, 463

Kava, preoperative evaluation of, 234

Keller arthroplasty, in diabetes mellitus, 787

Ketoacidosis, in diabetes mellitus, 639

Ketorolac, for perioperative pain, 260

Kidney function, preoperative evaluation of, 215

Koilonychia, 437

L

Lambotte, Albin, external fixation devices of, 2–3, 10

Lamotrigine, for diabetic neuropathy, 682

Lasegue's sign, 562

Lauge-Hansen classification, of foot and ankle trauma, 298

Leg, lower, deformities of. *See* Lower leg deformities.

Lepirudin, for deep venous thrombosis, 278–279

Leukocyte scan, in diabetic foot, 735–737

Leukonychia, 436

Levofloxacin, for diabetic foot infections, 659–660

Lidocaine
for diabetic neuropathy, 682
for preemptive analgesia, 246

Limb-length discrepancy
external fixation for, 20
footwear for, 597–598

Limb pressure measurements, in vascular disease, 693–695

Limb salvage
in diabetic foot, 794–797
in severe trauma, versus amputation, 301

Limberg (rhomboid) flaps, in diabetic foot reconstruction, 769

Linezolid, for diabetic foot infections, 659, 661

Lipid-lowering agents, preoperative evaluation of, 226

Lisfranc's fracture, malunion in, external fixation for, 47–49

Lithotripsy. *See* Extracorporeal shock wave therapy.

Liver function, preoperative evaluation of, 215

Local anesthesia, for preemptive analgesia, 243–248

Local random flaps, in diabetic foot reconstruction, 761–773

Long-term care, **383–394**
accidents in, 392
comprehensive plans for, 389
diabetic ulcers in, 387–388, 393–394
in home, 393–394
in nursing homes, 388–389
nutrition in, 391–392
pressure ulcers in, 384–387, 389–391
primary podiatric care in, 585–587
types of, 383

Lower leg deformities, external fixation correction of
anatomic considerations in, 120–124, 126, 129–136

devices for, 127, 129
malalignment evaluation in, 141–143
planning for, 136–143
rotational, 146–147, 150–154
short tibia, 144–145, 148–150
tibial angulation, 133, 145, 148
versus normal values, 137–141

Lower motor neuron lesions, assessment of, 562–563

LY333531, for diabetic neuropathy, 677

M

McGill Pain Questionnaire, 258

Macronychia, 432

Magnetic resonance imaging, in diabetic foot
in vascular evaluation, 701–702
with osteoarthropathy, 657, 737–738

Mal perforans ulcer. *See* Ulcer(s), in diabetes mellitus.

Malgaigne, Jean-Francois, external fixation devices of, 1, 10

Malnutrition
perioperative considerations in, 621
skin disorders in, 458–459

Malunion, external fixation for, 18–19, 47–49

Mangled Extremity Severity Score, 301

Medial plantar artery (instep) flaps, in diabetic foot reconstruction, 774

Medicamentosa dermatitis, 460

Medicare
class findings in, 414–415
codes of, 408–411
footwear provisions of, 593

Meglitinides, for diabetes mellitus, 643–644

Melatonin, for diabetic neuropathy, 679

Meperidine, for perioperative pain, 261

Meropenem, for diabetic foot infections, 664

Metabolic disorders, in diabetes mellitus, polyneuropathy in, 676–677

Metastasis, from cancer, 464

Metatarsal(s)
fractures of, external fixation for, 35, 168–170, 172–173
lesser, ulceration at, in diabetes mellitus, surgery for, 788–789
short, correction of, external fixation for, 36–39

Metatarsal bar, in footwear, 596–597

Metatarsalgia, 498–501

Metatarsocuneiform joint, first, arthrodesis of, external fixation for, 33–35

Metatarsophalangeal joint(s)
claw toe deformity involving, 489–491
first
arthrodesis of, external fixation for, 30–32
arthroplasty of, in diabetes mellitus, 786–787
hammertoe deformity involving, 487–491
lateral angulation of. *See* Hallux valgus.
rigidity of, 398, 491–493

Metformin, for diabetes mellitus, 222, 641–642, 644

N-Methyl-D-aspartate receptor antagonists, for preemptive analgesia, 250–251

Metronidazole, for diabetic foot infections, 662–664

Mexiletine, for diabetic neuropathy, 682

Micronychia, 432

Midfoot
external fixation applications in, **45–63**
angular deformity, 47–49
calcaneocuboid arthrodesis, 54–56
cavus osteotomy, 58–59
Charcot reconstruction. *See* Charcot foot and ankle.
devices for, 46
indications for, 46–47
naviculocuneiform arthrodesis, 57–58
osteomyelitis, 49–52, 59
talonavicular arthrodesis, 56–57
tarsometatarsal joint realignment and arthrodesis, 52–54
reconstruction of, in diabetes mellitus, 789

Miglitol, for diabetes mellitus, 221–222, 643

Minimum Data Set, for nursing home resident assessment, 388–390

Morphine
for perioperative pain, preemptive administration of, 249
for trauma, 299

Morton's neuroma, assessment of, 562

Motor function, assessment of, in elderly persons, 562–566

Motor neuropathy, in diabetes mellitus, 673

Multidisciplinary care, for elderly persons, 377–378

Muscle(s), evaluation of, in motor function assessment, 563–565

Muscle flaps, in diabetic foot reconstruction, 21–23, 775

N

Nafcillin, for diabetic foot infections, 659

Nail disorders
in diabetes mellitus
in elderly persons, 437
surgical treatment of, 785–786
in elderly persons, **431–442**
anonychia, 431
atrophy, 435–436
avulsion, 434–435
Beau's lines, 436
breaking, 437
congenital, 432
contusions, 434
dryness, 437
dystrophy, 436
exostosis, 434
foreign bodies, 435
growth changes, 433
heloma, 434, 445
hemorrhage, 434–435
hyperkeratosis, 434, 437
hyperpigmentation, 437
in diabetes mellitus, 437
in systemic diseases, 431–432, 437–438
inflammatory, 432
ingrown, 435
onycholysis, 431–432, 434–437
onychomycosis, 397, 433–434
onychophosis, 446
pain in, 397
psoriasis, 437
pterygium, 436–437
separation, 436
softening, 436
thickening, 435
treatment of, 585
warts, 432–433

Nateglinide, for diabetes mellitus, 221, 643–644

Naviculocuneiform joint, arthrodesis of, external fixation for, 57–58

Negative pressure therapy, for diabetic ulcers, 718

Neoplasia, of skin, in elderly persons, 463–464

Nerve(s)
cryotherapy effects on, 309
entrapment of, assessment of, 561–562
injury of, in external fixation, 92–93

Nerve blocks, for perioperative pain, 262–263
preemptive, 243–248
agents for, 246–247
duration of action of, 245
factors affecting, 244–245
mechanism of action of, 243–244
peripheral, 247

Nerve conduction studies, in diabetes mellitus, 675

Neuroarthropathy, Charcot. *See* Charcot foot and ankle.

Neurological evaluation
in ankle trauma, 296–297
in diabetes mellitus, 675, 713
of elderly persons, **547–571,** 616
formal examination in, 553–555
history in, 548–550
integrated sensorimotor function, 566–569
motor function, 562–566
observation in, 550–553
sensory function, 555–562
terminology of, 569–570

Neuroma, Morton's, assessment of, 562

Neuropathy. *See also* Peripheral neuropathy.
Charcot. *See* Charcot foot and ankle.
pain in, 399–400

Nikolsky's sign, 465

NMDA (N-methyl-D-aspartate) receptor antagonists, for preemptive analgesia, 250–251

Noncontact normothermic wound therapy, for diabetic ulcers, 718

Nonsteroidal anti-inflammatory drugs
for gout, 482
for osteoarthritis, 477
for perioperative pain, 250, 259–260
for rheumatoid arthritis, 479
preoperative evaluation of, 232

Nonunion
external fixation for, 18–19
extracorporeal shock wave therapy for, 332
in external fixation, 22

Norton Scale, for pressure ulcer staging, 385

Nortriptyline, for diabetic neuropathy, 680

NSAIDs. *See* Nonsteroidal anti-inflammatory drugs.

Numbness, in diabetic neuropathy, 673–674

Nursing homes, foot care in, 388–393

Nutrition
- assessment of, in amputation planning, 796
- for elderly persons, 458–459, 532
  - assessment of, 549
  - in long-term care, 391–392
  - surgical considerations in, 620–621

O

Obesity
- in osteoarthritis, 476
- preoperative evaluation of, 218

Occlusive vascular disease. *See* Arterial occlusive disease; Peripheral vascular disease.

Occupational disorders
- neurologic, 549
- skin, 460

Ofloxacin, for diabetic foot infections, 659–660, 664

Onychatrophia, 435–436

Onychauxis, 397, 432

Onychexallis, 433

Onychia, 432

Onychia punctata, 437

Onychia sicca, 437

Onychochauxis, 435

Onychoclasis, 437

Onychocryptosis, 435

Onychodystrophy, 436

Onychogryphosis, 397, 432

Onycholysis, 431–432, 434–437

Onychomadesis, 434–436

Onychomalacia, 434, 436

Onychomycosis, 397, 433–434

Onychophosis, 397, 434, 437, 446

Onychophyma, 433

Onychoptosis, 437

Onychorrhexis, 436

Onychoschizia, 436

Onychyphemia, 434–435

Open fractures, external fixation for, 15–16

Open reduction, in Charcot foot, 749, 751

Opioids
- for diabetic neuropathy, 679–680
- for perioperative pain, 249, 260–262

Oral antidiabetic agents, 220–222, 639–644

Orthofix external fixation system, for forefoot, 27–29

Orthoses. *See also* Footwear.
- for Charcot foot, 751
- for claw toes, 490
- for deformities, 523–526
- for diabetes mellitus, 576
- for hallux rigidus, 492–493
- for hallux valgus, 495–497
- for hammertoes, 490
- for metatarsalgia, 500–501
- for pes cavus, 505
- for pes planus, 503
- for plantar heel pain, 507–508
- for tailor's bunion, 497–498

Ossatron device, for plantar fasciitis, 326

Osteoarthritis
- in elderly persons
  - biomechanics of, 470–472
  - epidemiology of, 469–470
  - joints affected by, 472
  - pain in, 398
  - pathogenesis of, 474–475
  - surgery for, 609–610
  - treatment of, 472–477
- post-traumatic, ankle joint replacement for, case review of, **335–359**
- synovectomy for, external fixation after, 16

Osteoarthropathy, Charcot. *See* Charcot foot and ankle.

Osteomyelitis
- in diabetes mellitus
  - antibiotics for, 658–665
  - imaging in, 656–658, 729–740
  - of lesser metatarsals, 788
  - pathogens causing, 658
  - recommendations for, 665–666
  - surgery for, 665
  - treatment of, 718–719
  - versus Charcot foot, 746
- in elderly persons
  - in pressure ulcers, 386
  - in subungual abscess, 432
  - pain in, 399
- midfoot, external fixation for, 49–52, 59

Osteophytes, in osteoarthritis, 475

Osteoporosis
- pain in, 398
- preoperative considerations in, 613

Osteotomy
for cavus foot, external fixation for, 58–59
of metatarsals
external fixation of, 35–36
in diabetes mellitus, 788–789

Oxacillin, for diabetic foot infections, 659

Oximetry, in peripheral vascular disease, 539, 696–697

Oxycodone
for diabetic neuropathy, 679–680
for perioperative pain, 261

Oxygen therapy, for diabetic ulcers, 719

P

Pachonychia, 432

Pain. *See also* Pain management.
assessment of, 257–259
heel
in plantar fasciitis. *See* Plantar fasciitis.
retrocalcaneal exostectomy for, **361–366**
in arterial occlusive disease, 690
in diabetic neuropathy, 673–674, 678–683
in elderly persons, **395–406**
causes of, 395–396
impact of, 395–396
in arterial ulcers, 389
in arthritis, 398
in biomechanical disorders, 398
in diabetes mellitus, 398–399
in gout, 481–482
in hallux rigidus, 492
in hyperkeratosis, 397–398
in nail disorders, 397, 432, 434–435
in neurologic disorders, 399–400
in osteoarthritis, 476–477
in peripheral vascular disease, 399, 527–530
in pes cavus, 504–505
in systemic disease, 398
metatarsalgia, 498–501
perception of, assessment of, 558–559
plantar heel, 505–508
psychosocial correlates of, 400–401
skin changes in, 396–397
in external fixation, 22
physiology of, 237–240, 307–310

Pain management
in diabetic neuropathy, 678–683
in extracorporeal shock wave therapy, for plantar fasciitis, 329
in trauma, 298–299
postoperative, **257–267**
after return to home, 264–265
assessment in, 257–259
cryotherapy for, **307–322**
neural block in, 262–263
NSAIDs in, 259–260
opioids in, 260–261
patient-controlled analgesia in, 262
patient education in, 264
psychosocial issues in, 199–211
spinal/epidural analgesia in, 263–264

Parkhill, Clayton, external fixation devices of, 2, 10

Paronychia, 397

Paroxetine, for diabetic neuropathy, 681

Patient-controlled analgesia, for perioperative pain, 262

Pediatric patients, external fixation in, 22

Pedicle flaps, in diabetic foot reconstruction, 771, 773–779

Pemphigus vulgaris, 464–465

Pennig external fixation system, for forefoot, 27–28

Pentoxifylline, for diabetic neuropathy, 683

Percutaneous transluminal angioplasty, for vascular disease, in diabetes mellitus, 704

Peripheral neuropathy
in diabetes mellitus, **671–688**
amputation risk in, 783–784
classification of, 673–674
clinical course of, 674
definition of, 672
diagnosis of, 674–676
differential diagnosis of, 675–676
epidemiology of, 672–673
in elderly persons, 574–575, 578
pathology of, 676–677
treatment of, 677–683
ulcers in, 711
in elderly persons
diagnosis of, 379
flatfoot in, 502
in diabetes mellitus, 574–575, 578
types of, 554

Peripheral vascular disease. *See also* Arterial occlusive disease.
in elderly persons, **527–545**
diagnosis of, 379
healing ability and, 531–532

history of, 527–532
in diabetes mellitus, 575
noninvasive evaluation of, 539–543
pain in, 399
physical examination in, 532–538
risk factors for, 530–531
surgical risks in, 615–616
venous, 543–545

Peroneal bypass grafting, in diabetes mellitus, 703–704

Pes cavus, 503–505

Pes planus, 501–503

Phalanges, fractures of, external fixation for, 168–170, 172–173

Phenytoin, for diabetic neuropathy, 681

Photoplethysmography, in peripheral vascular disease, 539–541

Physical therapy
for ankle joint replacement, 340–341
for osteoarthritis, 476

Piezoelectric methods, for shock wave generation, 325–326

Pilon fractures, external fixation for, 15, 158, 160–164

Pioglitazone, for diabetes mellitus, 221, 642

Piperacillin, for diabetic foot infections, 664

Piperacillin/tazobactam, for diabetic foot infections, 660, 662–664

Plantar artery flaps, in diabetic foot reconstruction, 774

Plantar fasciitis, 505–508
conservative treatment of, 327–328
extracorporeal shock wave therapy for
adverse effects of, 329
approved devices for, 326
cautions with, 329
clinical studies of, 329–331
indications for, 328
procedure for, 329
fasciotomy for, 328
pathophysiology of, 327

Plantar keratosis, 447

Plate fixation, of ankle fractures, arthrosis after, joint replacement for, **335–359**

Platelet-derived growth factor gel, for diabetic ulcers, 717

Plethysmography, in peripheral vascular disease, 539–541

Plexopathy, 554

Podogeriatric care. *See* Elderly persons.

Polymicrobial infections, in diabetic foot, 658

Polyneuropathy, diabetic, 673–677

Polyol pathway, in diabetes mellitus, 677

Polyonychia, 432

Polypharmacy, in elderly persons, 376

Popliteal pulse, evaluation of, in peripheral vascular disease, 533–534

Porokeratosis plantaris discreta, 447

Poroma, eccrine, 446

Porphyria cutanea tarda, 465

Posterior tibial tendon dysfunction, 502

Postocclusive reactive hyperemia test, in peripheral vascular disease, 535–538

Posture, assessment of
in biomechanical evaluation, 515
in neurological evaluation, 550

Prednisone, preoperative evaluation of, 230

Preemptive analgesia, perioperative, **237–255**
benefits of, 242–243
clinical relevance of, 242–243
definition of, 242
goals of, 240–241
historical perspective of, 241
local, 243–248
misconceptions about, 241–242
multimodal, 251
NMDA receptor antagonists for, 250–251
NSAIDs for, 250
opioids for, 249
pain pathophysiology and, 237–240
preincisional versus postincisional block, 248
presurgical versus postsurgical block, 248

Preoperative evaluation, **213–235**
for diabetic foot elective procedures, 784–785
history-taking in, 213–217
laboratory testing in, 216–217
of medications, 219–234
anticoagulant, 226–229
antidepressant, 231
antidiabetic, 219–224
antiplatelet, 230
antipsychotic, 231
anxiolytic, 231
aspirin, 231–232
cardiovascular, 224–226

complementary, 232–234
corticosteroids, 230
NSAIDs, 231–232
risk factor assessment in, 217–219

Pressure relief, for diabetic ulcers, 718

Pressure Specifying Sensory Device, for sensory evaluation, 557–558

Pressure ulcers
in long-term care, 384–387, 389–391
assessment of, 384–385
prevention of, 389–390
risk for, 385, 390
staging of, 384–386
treatment of, 386–387, 391
postoperative, 624

Primary podiatric medicine, **583–591**
assessment in, 584
goals of, 586
in long-term care settings, 585–587
program for, 586–587
settings for, 584
standards of care in, 584
treatment in, 584–585

Probenecid, for diabetic foot infections, 659

Pronation
arthritis development in, 471
orthoses for, 525

Propranolol, preoperative evaluation of, 224–225

Proprioception, evaluation of, 559

Protein C, activated, resistance to, deep venous thrombosis in, 271

Protein S, defects of, deep venous thrombosis in, 271

Prothrombin, defects of, deep venous thrombosis in, 271

Psoriasis, 462–463

Psychiatric disorders, foot pain in, 401

Psychologic issues
in external fixation, 23–24
in foot pain, 400–401

Psychosocial management, of surgery patient, **199–211**
high-risk, 204
pretreatment screening, 200–201, 215
risk factor assessment and application in, 204–208
surgical outcome and, 201–204

Pterygium, of nail wall, 436–437

Pulmonary embolism, in deep venous thrombosis, 270–272, 274

Pulmonary function testing, preoperative, 214

Pulse, evaluation of
in diabetes mellitus, 713
in peripheral vascular disease, 533–534

Pulse volume recording, in peripheral vascular disease, 539, 695–696

Pump bump (Haglund's deformity), retrocalcaneal exostectomy for, **361–366**

Q

Quality of life, in foot pain, 400–401

Quantitative sensory testing, in diabetes mellitus, 675

Quinupristin-dalfopristin, for diabetic foot infections, 659, 662

R

Racial factors, in amputation, in diabetes mellitus, 799–800

Radiculopathy, 555

Radiography
in ankle trauma, 297–298
in diabetic foot, 656–657, 730–732

Ram's horn nails, 432

Random flaps, local, in diabetic foot reconstruction, 761–773

Rearfoot
alignment of, assessment of, 515–516
external fixation applications in, **65–96**
biomechanics of, 67–69
capabilities of, 66
circular, 67–69
complications of, 92–93
distraction arthrodiastasis, 90–92
frame removal in, 94
limitations of, 66–67
tibiocalcaneal arthrodesis, 16, 85–89
tibiotalar arthrodesis, 16, 74–85
triple arthrodesis, 16, 89–90
wire considerations in, 69–74
reconstruction of, in diabetes mellitus, 789–790

Reflexes, assessment of, 553, 566–568

Repaglinide, for diabetes mellitus, 221, 643–644

Resident Assessment Protocols, for nursing home residents, 388

Rest pain, in peripheral vascular disease, 530

Retrocalcaneal exostectomy, **361–366**

Reverse flow sural artery neurofasciocutaneous flaps, in diabetic foot reconstruction, 774–776

Rheumatoid arthritis
 in elderly persons, 477–481
  biomechanics of, 470–472
  diagnosis of, 477–478
  epidemiology of, 469
  joints affected by, 472
  pain in, 398
  treatment of, 472–474, 478–481
 subtalar arthrodesis in, external fixation for, 183–188

Rhomboid flaps, in diabetic foot reconstruction, 769–770, 772–773

Rifampicin, for diabetic foot infections, 660

Rigidity, in motor function assessment, 564

Risk factors
 for deep venous thrombosis, 269–270, 272–273
 preoperative evaluation of, 217–219
 psychosocial, assessment of, presurgical, 204–208

Road to Recovery pain assessment tool, 258–259

Rocker bar, in footwear, 597

Rockerbottom foot, external fixation for, 49–52

Rofecoxib, for perioperative pain, 250, 260

Romberg's test, 568–569

Ropivacaine, for preemptive analgesia, 246

Rosiglitazone, for diabetes mellitus, 221, 642, 644

Rotation flaps, in diabetic foot reconstruction, 764–765

S

Sagittal deformity, of midfoot, external fixation for, 49

Saint-John's wort, preoperative evaluation of, 233

Saline dressings, for diabetic ulcers, 717

Scintigraphy, in diabetic foot, 732–735
 with osteoarthropathy, 657
 with ulcers, 714–715

Screw fixation
 of ankle fractures, arthrosis after, joint replacement for, **335–359**
 of first metatarsocuneiform joint arthrodesis, external fixation with, 33–35

Sedation, in trauma, management of, 298–299

Seed corn (heloma miliare), 445

Segmental limb pressure measurements, in vascular disease, 693–695

Semmes-Weinstein monofilaments, for sensory evaluation, 556–557, 675, 713

Sensorimotor function, integrated, assessment of, 566–569

Sensory function, evaluation of
 in diabetes mellitus, 713
 in elderly persons, 555–562

Sensory neuropathy, in diabetes mellitus, 673

Sesamoidectomy, in diabetes mellitus, 787

Shank filler, in footwear, 597

Shock wave therapy, extracorporeal. *See* Extracorporeal shock wave therapy.

Shoes. *See* Footwear.

Skewfoot, external fixation for, 48–49

Skin, temperature of, in arterial occlusive disease, 691–692

Skin disorders
 in diabetes mellitus, examination of, 713–714
 in elderly persons, **453–467**
  aging changes and, 454, 459
  biopsy in, 454–456
  blistering, 464–465
  contact dermatitis, 460
  diagnosis of, 454–455
  in diabetes mellitus, 574–575
  in malnutrition, 458–459
  in peripheral vascular disease, 532–533
  in systemic disease, 453
  neoplastic, 463–464
  pain in, 396–397
  psoriasis, 462–463
  terminology of, 454–459
  ulcers. *See* Ulcer(s).
  warts, 432–433, 446–447, 464
  xerosis, 460, 462

Skin grafting, for diabetic foot, 759–761

Socks, for metatarsalgia, 499–500

Soft corn (heloma molle), 446

Soft tissue
contraction of, prevention of, external fixation in, 40
injury of, in external fixation, 21
reconstruction of, in diabetic foot, **757–781**
anatomic considerations in, 757–758
local random flaps in, 761–773
pedicle flaps in, 771, 773–779
skin grafting in, 759–761
team approach to, 757

Solid ankle cushion heel, in footwear, 597

Spasticity, in motor function assessment, 564

Spinal analgesia, cryotherapy effects on, 263–264

Spoon nails, 437

Staphylococcal infections, in diabetic foot, 658, 660–661

Stereognosia, assessment of, 558

Straight leg raising test, 562

Strength testing, in neurological evaluation, 564–566

Streptococcal infections, in diabetic foot, 658, 660–661

Stress, in hyperkeratosis formation, 444–445

Subpapillary venous plexus filling time test, in peripheral vascular disease, 534

Subtalar joint, arthrodesis of, external fixation for, **181–194**
case studies of, 185–194
in joint degeneration, 190–193
in rheumatoid arthritis, 185–190
indications for, 180
postoperative management in, 185
technique for, 182–185

Sudomotor axon reflex test, in diabetes mellitus, 675

Sulfonylureas, for diabetes mellitus, 220, 640–641, 644

Sulindac, for diabetic neuropathy, 679

Sural artery flaps, in diabetic foot reconstruction, 774–776

Surgery. *See also specific disorders and procedures.*
ankle joint replacement, **335–359**
cryotherapy after, **307–322**
deep venous thrombosis in. *See* Deep venous thrombosis.
extracorporeal shock wave, for plantar fasciitis, **323–334**
for diabetic foot
disease management in, 647–649
elective, **783–792**
Achilles tendon lengthening, 790
first ray, 786–787
goals of, 784
lesser digits, 785–786
lesser metatarsals, 788–789
midfoot, 789
nails, 785–786
preoperative evaluation for, 784–785
rearfoot, 789–790
in infections, 662–665
in ulceration, 720–721
for trauma, **291–306**
in elderly persons, **607–626**
age considerations in, 607
anesthesia for, 607
complications of, 623–624
for gout, 483
for osteoarthritis, 477
for rheumatoid arthritis, 480–481
goals of, 612
in peripheral vascular disease, 541–543
in primary care setting, 585
indications for, 608–612
perioperative care in, 621–622
postoperative care in, 622–623
preoperative assessment in, 619–621
risks of, 614–619
systems review for, 613–614
pain control in. *See* Pain management, postoperative.
preemptive analgesia for, **237–255**
preoperative evaluation and management for, **213–235**
psychosocial management in, **199–211**
retrocalcaneal exostectomy, **361–366**

Swelling, cryotherapy effects on, 309

Syme amputation, in diabetic foot, 797–798

Synovectomy, for osteoarthritis, external fixation after, 16

Synthes tubular external fixation, for subtalar arthrodesis, **181–194**
case studies of, 185–193
in joint degeneration, 191–193
in rheumatoid arthritis, 185–190
indications for, 182
postoperative management in, 185
technique for, 182–185

T

Tactile Circumferential Discriminator, for sensory evaluation, 557

Tailor's bunion, in elderly persons, 497–498

Talonavicular joint, arthrodesis of, external fixation for, 56–57

Talus, fractures of, external fixation for, 160, 162–166, 169

Tarsometatarsal joint, arthrodesis of, external fixation for, 52–54

Temperature sensation, assessment of, 559–560

Terry's nails, 437

Tetanus, in ankle trauma, 294–295

Thiazolidinediones, for diabetes mellitus, 221, 642

Thomas heel, in footwear, 597

Thrombosis, venous. *See also* Deep venous thrombosis.
 in elderly persons, 544–545, 616

Tibia
 angulation of, external fixation correction of, 133, 145, 148
 deformities of. *See* Lower leg deformities.
 fractures of, joint replacement for, case review of, **335–359**
 pilon fractures of, external fixation for, 15, 160, 162–166
 rotational deformity of, external fixation correction of, 146–147, 150–154
 short, external fixation correction of, 144–145, 148–150

Tibial pulse, posterior, evaluation of, in peripheral vascular disease, 533–534

Tibiocalcaneal joint, arthrodesis of, external fixation for, 16, 85–89

Tibiotalar joint, arthrodesis of, external fixation for, 16, 74–85

Ticarcillin/clavulanate, for diabetic foot infections, 662–664

Ticlopidine, preoperative evaluation of, 230

Tinazaprin, for deep venous thrombosis, 278

Tinea unguium, pain in, 397

Tinel's sign, 562

Toe(s)
 alignment of, assessment of, 516–517
 claw, 489–491
 deformities of, in diabetes mellitus, surgical treatment of, 785–786
 gout in, 398, 481–483
 great. *See subjects starting with* Hallux.
 hammer deformity of, 487–491, 785–786
 heloma of. *See* Heloma.
 pressure measurements in, in vascular disease, 695
 tailor's bunion of, 497–498

Tolazamide, for diabetes mellitus, 640–641

Tolbutamide, for diabetes mellitus, 640–641

Topiramate, for diabetic neuropathy, 682

Total-contact cast, for diabetic ulcers, 718

Touch, evaluation of, 556–558

Tourniquet, for trauma repair, 301

Tramadol, for diabetic neuropathy, 680

Trandolapril, for diabetic neuropathy, 683

Transcutaneous electrical nerve stimulation, for diabetic neuropathy, 683

Transcutaneous oximetry, in peripheral vascular disease, 539, 696–697

Transposition flaps, in diabetic foot reconstruction, 764–766

Trauma. *See also* Fracture(s).
 arthrosis after, ankle joint replacement for, case review of, **335–359**
 external fixation for, **159–180**
  ankle arthrodesis, 166–169
  ankle joint bridging, 160, 162–166
  calcaneal fractures, 169–170
  contractures, 176, 178
  Ilizarov technique for, 172–173, 176–179
  metatarsal fractures, 170–172, 174–175
  phalangeal fractures, 169–172, 174–175
  talar fractures, 169
 in diabetes mellitus, ulcers in, 711
 perioperative management of, **291–306**
  dressings in, 303–304
  historical perspective of, 292–293
  history taking in, 294–295
  in displaced fracture, 302
  in open injury, 299–302
  initial evaluation in, 293
  internal fixation in, 302–303
  pain control in, 298–299
  physical examination in, 295–298
  surgical procedure in, 299–305
  systematic evaluation in, 294–298
  wound closure in, 303

Tremor, assessment of, in neurological evaluation, 550–551

Tricyclic antidepressants
for diabetic neuropathy, 680–681
preoperative evaluation of, 231

Triple arthrodesis, external fixation for, 16, 89–90

Tuning fork, for vibratory sensation assessment, 560–561

Two-point discrimination test, for sensory evaluation, 557–558

Tyloma (callus), 397–398, 445

U

Ulcer(s)
in diabetes mellitus, **709–728**. *See also* Ulcer(s), in elderly persons, in diabetes mellitus.
classification of, 715
epidemiology of, 710
etiology of, 711–712
evaluation of, 712–715
prevention of, 721–722. *See also* Surgery, for diabetic foot, elective.
risk factors for, 783–784
treatment of
healing promotion modalities in, 715–719
surgical, 720–721
in elderly persons, 465–466
arterial, 389
in diabetes mellitus
assessment of, 573–582
in long-term care, 387–388, 393–394
pain in, 399
prevention of, 573–582
pressure, in long-term care, 384–387, 389–391
treatment of, 466
venous stasis, 388–389
pressure. *See* Pressure ulcers.

Ultrasonography
Duplex
in deep venous thrombosis, 274–275
in peripheral vascular disease, 697–699
in Charcot foot, in diabetes mellitus, 657–658

University of Texas, wound classification system of, 715

Upper motor neuron lesions, assessment of, 563

Urate deposition, in gout, 481–483

Urticaria, 460

V

V-Y advancement flap, in diabetic foot reconstruction, 763–764

Vacuum-assisted closure, of diabetic ulcers, 718

Valerian, preoperative evaluation of, 234

Valgus deformity, of midfoot, external fixation for, 48–49

Valproate, for diabetic neuropathy, 683

Vancomycin, for diabetic foot infections, 659–661, 664

Varus deformity, of midfoot, external fixation for, 48–49

Vascular examination, in ankle trauma, 295–296

Vasculopathy, in diabetes mellitus
polyneuropathy in, 676–677
ulcers in, 711

Vena cava, inferior, interruption therapy for, for deep venous thrombosis, 280

Venography, in deep venous thrombosis, 275

Venous disease, in elderly persons, 543–545
stasis ulcers, 388–389
surgical risks in, 616

Venous stasis, deep venous thrombosis in, 270–271

Venous thrombosis, deep. *See* Deep venous thrombosis.

Verrucae. *See* Warts.

Vibratory sensation, assessment of, 560–561

W

Wagner Scale, for diabetic ulcer staging, 387

Warfarin
for deep venous thrombosis, 279
preoperative evaluation of, 227–228

Warts, in elderly persons, 446–447
of nail area, 432–433
treatment of, 464

Wedges, in footwear, 595–596

Whartenberg pinwheel, in pain perception assessment, 558

Wires, in external fixation
of first metatarsocuneiform joint arthrodesis, 33–35
of first metatarsophalangeal joint arthrodesis, 30–32
of rearfoot procedures, 69–74

Wound. *See also* Ulcer(s).
assessment of, in diabetic ulcers, 714–715
treatment of, in pressure ulcers, 386–387

X

Xerosis, 460, 462

Z

Z-plasty, in double-Z rhomboid flaps, in diabetic foot reconstruction, 769–770, 772–773

Zolpidem, for diabetic neuropathy, 679

United States Postal Service

Statement of Ownership, Management, and Circulation

1. Publication Title	2. Publication Number	3. Filing Date
Clinics in Podiatric Medicine and Surgery	0 8 9 1 - 8 4 2 2	9/15/02
4. Issue Frequency	5. Number of Issues Published Annually	6. Annual Subscription Price
Jan, Apr, Jul, Oct	4	$148.00

7. Complete Mailing Address of Known Office of Publication (*Not printer*) (*Street, city, county, state, and ZIP+4*)

Elsevier Science
6277 Sea Harbor Drive, Orlando, FL 32887-4800, Orange County

Contact Person: Amy Snyder

Telephone: 215-238-8319

8. Complete Mailing Address of Headquarters or General Business Office of Publisher (*Not printer*)

Elsevier Science, The Curtis Center, Independence Square West, Philadelphia, PA 19106-3399

9. Full Names and Complete Mailing Addresses of Publisher, Editor, and Managing Editor (*Do not leave blank*)

Publisher (*Name and complete mailing address*)

Glen Campbell, Elsevier Science, The Curtis Center, Independence Square West, Philadelphia, PA 19106-3399

Editor (*Name and complete mailing address*)

Karen Sorensen, Elsevier Science, The Curtis Center, Independence Square West, Philadelphia, PA 19106-3399

Managing Editor (*Name and complete mailing address*)

Heather Cullen, Elsevier Science, The Curtis Center, Independence Square West, Philadelphia, PA 19106-3399

10. Owner (*Do not leave blank. If the publication is owned by a corporation, give the name and address of the corporation immediately followed by the names and addresses of all stockholders owning or holding 1 percent or more of the total amount of stock. If not owned by a corporation, give the names and addresses of the individual owners. If owned by a partnership or other unincorporated firm, give its name and address as well as those of each individual owner. If the publication is published by a nonprofit organization, give its name and address.*)

Full Name	Complete Mailing Address
Wholly owned subsidiary of	4520 East-West Highway
Reed/Elsevier, US holdings	Bethesda, MD 20814

11. Known Bondholders, Mortgagees, and Other Security Holders Owning or Holding 1 Percent or More of Total Amount of Bonds, Mortgages, or Other Securities. If none, check box ► None

Full Name	Complete Mailing Address
N/A	

12. Tax Status (*For completion by nonprofit organizations authorized to mail at nonprofit rates*) (*Check one*)
The purpose, function, and nonprofit status of this organization and the exempt status for federal income tax purposes:
Has Not Changed During Preceding 12 Months
Has Changed During Preceding 12 Months (*Publisher must submit explanation of change with this statement*)

(*See Instructions on Reverse*)

13. Publication Title Clinics in Podiatric Medicine and Surgery			14. Issue Date for Circulation Data Below April 2002	
15. **Extent and Nature of Circulation**			**Average No. Copies Each Issue During Preceding 12 Months**	**No. Copies of Single Issue Published Nearest to Filing Date**
a. Total Number of Copies (*Net press run*)			2550	2300
b. Paid and/or Requested Circulation	(1)	Paid/Requested Outside-County Mail Subscriptions Stated on Form 3541. (*Include advertiser's proof and exchange copies*)	1652	1557
	(2)	Paid In-County Subscriptions Stated on Form 3541 (*Include advertiser's proof and exchange copies*)		
	(3)	Sales Through Dealers and Carriers, Street Vendors, Counter Sales, and Other Non-USPS Paid Distribution	111	88
	(4)	Other Classes Mailed Through the USPS		
c. Total Paid and/or Requested Circulation [*Sum of 15b. (1), (2), (3), and (4)*] ►			1763	1645
d. Free Distribution by Mail (*Samples, compliment-ary, and other free*)	(1)	Outside-County as Stated on Form 3541	72	74
	(2)	In-County as Stated on Form 3541		
	(3)	Other Classes Mailed Through the USPS		
e. Free Distribution Outside the Mail (*Carriers or other means*)				
f. Total Free Distribution (*Sum of 15d. and 15e.*) ►			72	74
g. Total Distribution (*Sum of 15c. and 15f.*) ►			1835	1719
h. Copies not Distributed			715	581
i. Total (*Sum of 15g. and h.*) ►			2550	2300
j. Percent Paid and/or Requested Circulation (*15c. divided by 15g. times 100*)			96%	96%

16. Publication of Statement of Ownership

Publication required. Will be printed in the **October 2002** issue of this publication. Publication not required

17. Signature and Title of Editor, Publisher, Business Manager, or Owner	Date
Jean M. Fanucci Jean M. Fanucci, Director of Subscription Services	9/15/02

I certify that all information furnished on this form is true and complete. I understand that anyone who furnishes false or misleading information on this form or who omits material or information requested on the form may be subject to criminal sanctions (including fines and imprisonment) and/or civil sanctions (including civil penalties).

Instructions to Publishers

1. Complete and file one copy of this form with your postmaster annually on or before October 1. Keep a copy of the completed form for your records.
2. In cases where the stockholder or security holder is a trustee, include in items 10 and 11 the name of the person or corporation for whom the trustee is acting. Also include the names and addresses of individuals who are stockholders who own or hold 1 percent or more of the total amount of bonds, mortgages, or other securities of the publishing corporation. In item 11, if none, check the box. Use blank sheets if more space is required.
3. Be sure to furnish all circulation information called for in item 15. Free circulation must be shown in items 15d, e, and f.
4. Item 15h., Copies not Distributed, must include (1) newsstand copies originally stated on Form 3541, and returned to the publisher, (2) estimated returns from news agents, and (3), copies for office use, leftovers, spoiled, and all other copies not distributed.
5. If the publication had Periodicals authorization as a general or requester publication, this Statement of Ownership, Management, and Circulation must be published; it must be printed in any issue in October or, if the publication is not published during October, the first issue printed after October.
6. In item 16, indicate the date of the issue in which this Statement of Ownership will be published.
7. Item 17 must be signed.

Failure to file or publish a statement of ownership may lead to suspension of Periodicals authorization.

Changing Your Address?

Make sure your subscription changes too! When you notify us of your new address, you can help make our job easier by including an exact copy of your Clinics label number with your old address (see illustration below.) This number identifies you to our computer system and will speed the processing of your address change. Please be sure this label number accompanies your old address and your corrected address—you can send an old Clinics label with your number on it or just copy it exactly and send it to the address listed below.

We appreciate your help in our attempt to give you continuous coverage. Thank you.

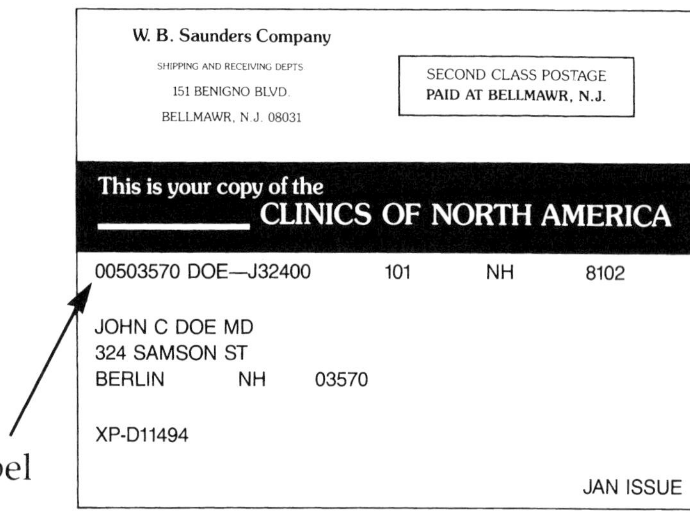
W. B. Saunders Company
SHIPPING AND RECEIVING DEPTS
151 BENIGNO BLVD.
BELLMAWR, N.J. 08031

SECOND CLASS POSTAGE
PAID AT BELLMAWR, N.J.

This is your copy of the
________ CLINICS OF NORTH AMERICA

00503570 DOE—J32400 101 NH 8102

JOHN C DOE MD
324 SAMSON ST
BERLIN NH 03570

XP-D11494

JAN ISSUE

Your Clinics Label Number

Copy it exactly or send your label along with your address to:
W.B. Saunders Company, Customer Service
Orlando, FL 32887-4800
Call Toll Free 1-800-654-2452

Please allow four to six weeks for delivery of new subscriptions and for processing address changes.